THE TWO PILLARS POWER PACK 2 IN 1

REIN IN YOUR PHYSICAL AND MENTAL HEALTH TO
SUPERCHARGE YOUR LIFE IN LESS THAN 7 DAYS + 10
LIFE ALTERING STEPS TO CONFRONT BODY
IMAGE ANXIETY AND EATING DISORDERS

B&V HEALTHY LIVING

ABOUT THE AUTHOR

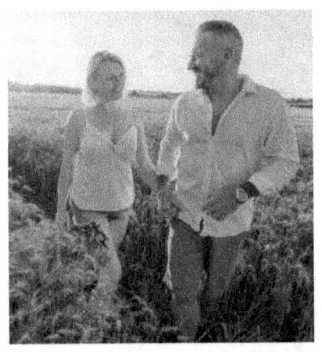 Brian and Vanda of B&V Healthy Living are passionate about helping people improve their quality of life. They endorse an organic lifestyle centered around European practices like growing your own fruit and vegetables, walking and biking, connecting with nature, and eating a healthy and balanced diet. Vanda promotes a healthy and happy mindset of daily affirmations, self-care and self-love, healthy eating, banishing negativity and focusing on positivity, and improving mental health. Throughout their marriage, they have experienced life's ups and downs, the many changes and challenges that the modern world presents, and have combined their knowledge and growth to create a motivational and inspirational company that helps people to live with positivity, purpose, and good health. Check out their blog and find out more about them at **www.bvhealthyliving.com**.

CONTENTS

INTRODUCTION: REIN IN YOUR PHYSICAL AND MENTAL HEALTH TO SUPERCHARGE YOUR LIFE IN LESS THAN 7 DAYS..................................13

1. THE TWO PILLARS: A PERFECT PARTNERSHIP.....................17
   WHAT IS MENTAL HEALTH?..18
   WHAT IS PHYSICAL HEALTH?..24
   THE MENTAL AND PHYSICAL CONNECTION 30
   INTERACTIVE ELEMENT: HEALTH INVENTORY 33

2. NOURISHING YOURSELF THE RIGHT WAY 39
   WHAT IS NUTRITION? 40
   THE DANGERS OF DIET CULTURE 43
   HOW DIET IMPACTS HEALTH...46
   STEPS TO IMPROVING YOUR DIET.....................................48
   INTERACTIVE ELEMENT: EVALUATE YOUR EATING HABITS 52

3. MOVING TOWARD HEALTH...55
   WHY DOES EXERCISE MATTER?..57
   EXERCISE AND MENTAL HEALTH......................................59
   EXERCISING FOR BEGINNERS 61
   FINDING TIME FOR FITNESS 65
   INTERACTIVE ELEMENT: EXERCISE CHART 68

4. A RESTFUL APPROACH 71
   THE SCIENCE OF SLEEP 72
   SLEEP AND HEALTH...74
   SLEEP HYGIENE..75
   INTERACTIVE ELEMENT: SET YOUR SLEEP SCHEDULE 81

5. SAYING "BYE" TO BAD HABITS 83
   DEFINING GOOD AND BAD HABITS 84
   BREAKING BAD HABITS 89
   GROWING GOOD HABITS 92
   INTERACTIVE ELEMENT: BREAK A BAD HABIT!...............96

6. THE SELF-AWARE CHAMPION 101

WHAT IS SELF-AWARENESS? 102

THE POWER OF SELF-AWARENESS ON THE PILLARS 106

HOW TO DEVELOP YOUR SELF-AWARENESS 108

INTERACTIVE ELEMENT: THE SELF- AWARENESS
WORKSHEET 111

7. MOVING THE GOAL POST 115

GOAL POWER 116

SETTING SMART GOALS 118

MY GOAL FAILED... NOW WHAT? 123

INTERACTIVE ELEMENT: SET A SMART GOAL! 127

8. KEEPING A HEALTHY HOME 131

YOUR HOME AND YOUR HEALTH 132

MAKE YOUR HOME A SANCTUARY 136

INTERACTIVE ELEMENT: YOUR ROOM-BY- ROOM DEEP
CLEAN CHECKLIST 143

9. A NEAT 7-DAY PACKAGE 149

ROUTINES 151

BUILDING THE BEST ROUTINE FOR THE BEST YOU 160

CONCLUSION 169

REFERENCES 175

Introduction: 10 LIFE-ALTERING STEPS TO CONFRONT BODY IMAGE
ANXIETY AND EATING DISORDERS - 185

1. Step 1 - Acknowledging the Struggle 191

Anxiety and Body Dysmorphia 192

The Impact of Body Dysmorphia 197

2. Step 2 - Breaking the Silence and Seeking Help 207

Eating Disorders 209

Seeking Help 215

Stigma and Support..218
Help Resources 221
Step 2 Activity: Open Up...223

3. Step 3 - Cultivating Self- Compassion and Mindfulness....................227
Developing Self-Compassion 228
Managing Anxiety and Negativity with Mindfulness..................231
Self-Awareness for Healing..234
Step 3 Activity: Guided Self- Compassion Exercises 236

4. Step 4 - Unraveling Negative Thought Patterns......................................243
The Connection Between Thoughts, Emotions, and Behavior................244
Cognitive Behavioral Therapy..246
Journaling and Cognitive Reframing Exercises...........................250
Step 4 Activity: Positive Journaling..252

5. Step 5 - Nourishing Your Body and Mind 255
The Physical/Mental Health Connection....................................256
Establishing Healthy Eating Habits 259
Exercise for Your Mental Well-Being 265
Step 5 Activity: Mindful Eating Practice 269

6. Step 6 - Identifying and Coping With Triggers 271
What Are Triggers?...272
Identifying Your Triggers...275
Coping Strategies..278
Step 6 Activity: Trigger Journal...282

7. Step 7 - Embracing Body Acceptance and Positivity 285
The Power of Body Positivity..286
Practicing Body Positivity 289
Step 7 Activity: Create Your Body Positivity Collage................294

8. Step 8 - Practicing Self- Care and Self-Love 297
Self-Care and Body Image Issues...297
Self-Care Activities..298
Cultivate Self-Love and Compassion 304

Setting Boundaries and Saying No...306
Step 8 Activity: Create Your Self-Care Routine...................................314

9. Step 9 - Fostering Resilience and Growth......................................317
Resilience and Body Dysmorphia..318
How to Build Your Resilience...320
Developing a Growth Mindset..324
Step 9 Activity: Resilience Reflection..327

10. Step 10 - Embracing a Life of Purpose and Fulfillment....................329
Discovering Your Personal Values and Passions 330
Step 10 Activity: Your Life Vision Board 346

Conclusion 349
References 353

JUST FOR YOU!

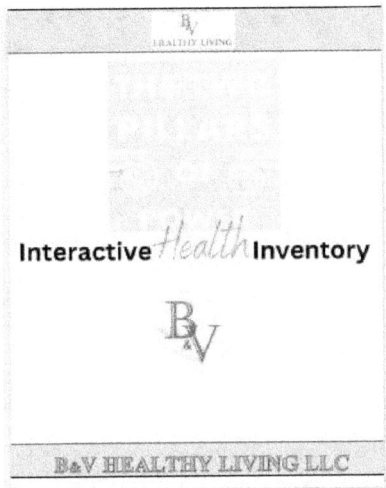

Interactive *Health* Inventory

B&V

B&V HEALTHY LIVING LLC

A FREE GIFT TO OUR READERS
Download and print the **Two Pillars of Power:**
Interactive Health Inventory

The Health Inventory should be used as you progress
through each chapter assessing your current health and
setting new goals that will transform your life right away!
Visit the link:

https://bvhealthyliving.org/HealthInventory

THE TWO PILLARS OF POWER

REIN IN YOUR PHYSICAL AND MENTAL HEALTH TO SUPERCHARGE YOUR LIFE IN LESS THAN 7 DAYS

B&V HEALTHY LIVING

INTRODUCTION

When you think of the two pillars, picture them as two narrow columns of stone, like those of the ancient temples in Greece, still standing today after thousands of years of war and weather. Imagine you stand atop them, with a foot planted on each. When the pillars are weak, they are prone to breaking, falling, and swaying at the slightest hurricane of life. If one sways or topples, you'll be left flailing, likely to fall, and no matter how strong the other is, it cannot hold you alone. When they are both strong, they will support you through your decisions, pursuits, and adventures, and you can pursue your dreams and goals with surety, knowing you have a solid foundation for growth. So, what are the two pillars?

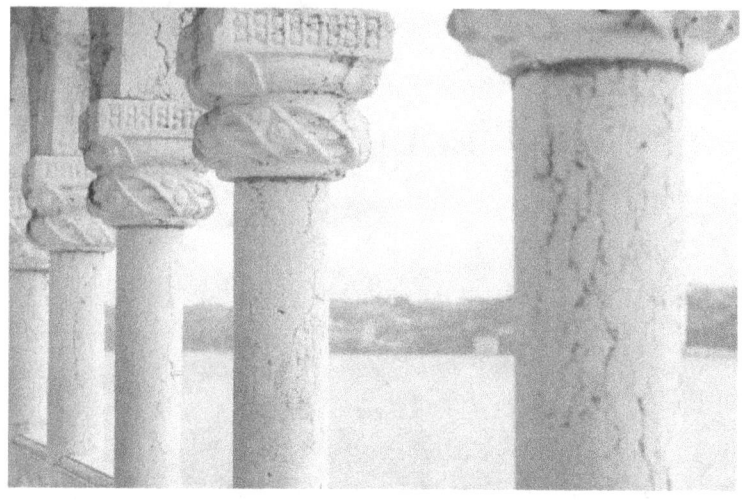

Mental and physical health are the two columns upon which your whole life depends. The deep-rooted connection between them has the power to alter your life for both good and bad. Your mental health and mind are the power behind focus, effort, ambition, and emotion, while your physical health and body are the tools that allow you to pursue adventure and the milestones of life. Both require great care and attention to live up to their full potential and provide optimal support throughout your life. The connection between them runs deep in our cells, nerves, hormones, and chemicals, rippling through our bodies in our blood. When one suffers, the other suffers too—a healthy body requires a healthy mind, and vice versa. Perhaps this has brought you to this book. You can feel that your pillars are imbalanced, that you are flailing and in need of support. You recognize that something about how you have been living your life isn't working in the best interests of your health, ambitions, or happiness, and you are looking to change that. This is the first, all-important step in the journey to come. Finding the energy and motivation to make the change you need in life.

This catalyst for change comes when you cannot stand the idea of going on the way you have been when you believe you deserve better. Many people struggle with mental health to the point they cannot leave the house, keep a job, sustain a healthy diet, or cannot form healthy relation-ships. People with physical health issues can find they have no energy or ability to socialize, work, clean, or exer-cise. Alongside pain and illness, they can easily develop mental health problems. In almost every success story, there has been a moment of clarity about the situation, an overwhelming desire to make positive change, and a need to break the negative cycle and take back control of life and health. This is that point.

This is the beginning of your success story, and like the others who have succeeded, you will turn your life around and find purpose, joy, health, and vitality again. With this book, you can rebuild your life, pursue your dreams and ambitions, and feel energized and healthy, well-rested and focused. You can get up and face the world, take control of your future, and forge a path of positivity.

Of course, lasting and positive change doesn't happen overnight. It takes dedication and discipline every day to rein in your life and take back control of it, to undo the bad habits and routines, to dispel the doubts and distractions, but with this book as your guide, you have the opportunity to make an incredible difference to your life in just a week. You'll be given an in-depth understanding of the two pillars of mental and physical health, plus information and exercises on eating right for your body, finding time for fitness, encouraging replenishing sleep, overcoming mental health roadblocks, building good habits and routines, and much more. Interactive activities will help you to focus your efforts and self-reflect on your needs and progress, and by the end of the book, you will have learned skills and built habits that you can harness to change your life in just one supercharged week. That incredible week starts right now, from the moment you turn this page and begin your journey to a fulfilling and happy life. Let's get started!

THE TWO PILLARS: A PERFECT PARTNERSHIP

"A fit body, a calm mind, a house full of love. These things cannot be bought – they must be earned."

— NAVAL RAVIKANT

The key to a perfect partnership is balance, mutual support, and an understanding of each person's pivotal role in the partnership—the same is valid for mental and physical health. Everyone strives to be happy and healthy in mind and body. Still, without understanding the deep connection between the two pillars, it is easy to fall into habits that favor one or the other and, in doing so, unbalance everything. An awareness of how your mental and physical health intertwines will encourage you to make informed and effective choices about your health and help you to view yourself with empathy and your problems with clarity.

WHAT IS MENTAL HEALTH?

Mental health encompasses our emotional and psychological states, as well as our personal and social well-being. It plays a vital part in how we act, react, think, feel, and approach the world, from solving problems and dealing with stress, conflict, and emotions to showing empathy for and understanding others. Mental health influences our thoughts and actions throughout our lives, and it constantly changes and evolves as we experience and learn more about ourselves and the world. A healthy mind with a positive mindset is vital to enjoying life, being successful in your endeavors, supercharging your self-confidence, and achieving your goals, while poor mental health can prevent you from pursuing your ambitions and reaching your full potential—this is why mental health is one of the two vital pillars of life. Struggling with mental health is nothing to be ashamed of—almost everyone you meet is struggling in some way—but by recognizing the negative impact it can have on your life and working to take back control of your mind to find purpose and happiness again, is the most extraordinary act of kindness you can do yourself.

Factors That Impact Mental Health

Our minds are complex and advanced, and every single decision you make, and everything that happens to you has an impact on you and your mental health. Some experiences will strengthen, others may harm, and you must find ways to maintain a positive mindset to progress through life. Someone in a state of good, strong mental health is better equipped to face challenges and form connections than someone who is struggling with theirs, which highlights the importance of working to improve your mindset. There are many factors that contribute to mental health problems, almost all of which are negative experiences forced on us throughout our lives that damage our sense of self and self-worth and force us to question or relinquish control over our lives. These factors include isolation and loneliness, childhood abuse and neglect, trauma, discrimination, bullying, domestic violence, and grief, all of which can have lasting impacts on children and adults. Economic disadvantages like unemployment, poverty, debt, and homelessness also damage our mental health, as does severe or long-term stress and addiction.

Lifestyle factors such as diet, lack of sleep, work, and drugs can also lead to struggles with mental health, although more often, they are part of a more significant problem. While you should seek professional help and treatment for mental health problems, it is also essential to rule out any potential physical causes first to ensure you get the help you really need.

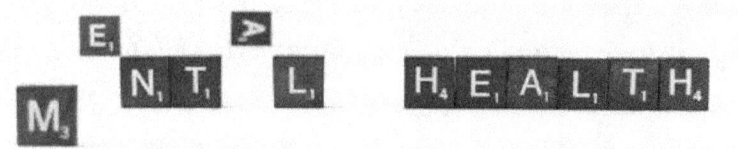

Mental Health Disorders

Mental health disorders and illnesses are more common than many people realize. In the United States, it is estimated that more than one in five adults are living with mental illnesses of some kind, including behavioral and emotional disorders (National Institute of Mental Health, 2023). Millions of people live every day with any number or variety of mental disorders, from manageable to severe, and understanding the different and most common types will help you to recognize them in yourself and in others, meaning you can better understand yourself and your needs, and practice empathy with others.

Anxiety

There are multiple forms of anxiety, none of which is just feeling scared. Anxiety can be far more debilitating than the short bursts of fear and nervousness we are supposed to feel in times of stress. Instead, people with anxiety experience excessive and prolonged fear and worry, often without an obvious or immediate cause, which can seriously impact their everyday functioning. People can experience anxiety throughout their lives, from childhood to adulthood, and can struggle to make friends, progress in education and employment, and form healthy relationships. Some of the many varieties of anxiety are general anxiety disorder, panic disorder, social anxiety, and separation anxiety.

Depression

Depression, a common and severe mental disorder, is characterized by long-term feelings of sadness, emptiness, and irritability, often combined with a lack of energy and interest, loss of pleasure in things, poor concentration and memory, feeling guilty, worthless, or hopeless, and experiencing suicidal or morbid thoughts. Physically, a depressed person may feel constantly tired, have trouble sleeping, experience weight and appetite fluctuations, and frequent headaches and pains. There are effective treatments available for depression, including psychotherapy and, in some instances, medication.

Bipolar Disorder

This mental disorder causes alternating mood, activity, and energy shifts, switching between depressive and manic episodes. Symptoms include "up" periods of feeling elated, impulsive, highly energized, and irritable to "down" periods of indifference, hopelessness, and other depressive behavior. These episodes can last days or weeks at a time and tend to go through cycles. Long-term treatment is usually necessary to manage bipolar disorders.

PTSD

Post Traumatic Stress Disorder manifests after exposure to a traumatic event that is often horrific and threatening. PTSD is most often characterized by re-living the event (in flashbacks, nightmares, and intrusive memories), avoiding thoughts, memories, people, and situations that remind the sufferer of the event, and experiencing persistent feelings of threat. Symptoms can last from weeks up to years and have a catastrophic impact on daily life— luckily, there are effective psychological treatment options.

Schizophrenia

This serious disorder affects how a person feels, thinks, behaves, and perceives the world. Symptoms include psychotic episodes with hallucinations, delusions, and noticeable thought and movement disorders. Other symptoms can appear similar to depression and other mental illnesses, like struggling to concentrate, plan, or take interest, and trouble with memory and decision-making. People with schizophrenia are not often violent to others. Still, they can be a danger to themselves, and treatment is essential to help them manage the condition and improve their ability to function in daily life.

Eating Disorders

The most common eating disorders are anorexia, bulimia, and binge-eating disorder. These are not simply diet or lifestyle choices. They are serious illnesses that impact behavior, thought, and emotions and harm the body. People suffering from anorexia and bulimia may avoid or severely restrict food, weigh themselves frequently or obsessively, and be unable to see themselves as anything other than "overweight" no matter how they look. They may purge food by vomiting, exercise excessively, and even use laxatives. Binge-eating disorder is characterized by a loss of control over eating. The person may consume large amounts of food in short periods of time, eat when they're not hungry, feel guilty or ashamed about eating, and hide food to eat in secret. They are likely to be over-weight or obese and struggle to lose weight even when dieting. Eating disorders can be managed and treated with psychotherapy and medication.

Disruptive Behavior and Dissocial Disorders

Symptoms of these disorders usually, but not always, manifest in childhood and include persistent problems with behavior, defiance, disobedience, and conduct that violates others' fundamental rights and societal norms and rules. Treatment usually involves parents and teachers and cognitive and social skills training.

Neurodevelopmental Disorders

Neurodevelopmental Disorders develop during childhood and adolescence and affect cognitive and behavioral development, often resulting in problems with motor skills, language and understanding, and social skills. There is a wide range of disorders in this area, some very manageable, others more serious. Some common ones are Attention Deficit Hyperactivity Disorder (ADHD), autism spectrum disorder, and intellectual development disorders.

WHAT IS PHYSICAL HEALTH?

Maintaining good physical health is crucial for your well-being, quality of life, and your view of yourself. Physical health encompasses your fitness level and your body's ability to fight disease and work at peak function to support you through life. There are many benefits to having good physical health, including having more energy, living longer, being better equipped to fight illness, getting a better night's sleep, and being able to enjoy active pursuits. For many people, having good physical health enables them to feel strong and confident in their body and gives them peace of mind knowing they look after themselves. Working to strengthen your body and care for yourself also helps you better understand your body and its needs so you can recognize the symptoms and warning signs of disease earlier.

Factors That Impact Physical Health

As with mental health, there are many external and internal factors that affect our physical health and our ability to look after ourselves. You have control over some elements, like diet, lifestyle, and physical activity, whereas you cannot control others, like age and genetics. Lifestyle choices such as diet, exercise, and what you eat and drink and put into your body (including alcohol and smoking) have a powerful effect on the body, as do environmental factors like sun exposure or proximity to harmful substances. Your human biology (genetics and physiology) plays a crucial part, with factors making it easier or harder to maintain and achieve good physical health. Access to good healthcare is another vital factor, and regular check-ups and quick treatments can substantially impact your body's health.

Physical Health Disorders

The body is very complex and, as such, finds itself vulnerable to illnesses and diseases at every stage of life, no matter how healthy or careful you are. Unlike mental health disorders, physical disorders can be evident and have a noticeable impact on your daily life. While keeping healthy can prevent illnesses from causing long-term damage or even death, it is always best to be aware of the dangers and symptoms of some common physical health disorders. Hence, you are able to recognize them quickly and understand the problem. Symptoms can appear suddenly or grow slowly over time, so frequent check-ups can be instrumental, especially if you have a family history of medical conditions.

Cancer

One of the most common health conditions in the world, cancer occurs when cells grow uncontrollably and spread to areas of the body where they don't belong. There are many forms of cancer as these cells can and will grow anywhere in the body, but some of the most prevalent cancers are lung, breast, skin, prostate, and stomach. While cancer can be frightening, the earlier it is diagnosed, the better, and more treatments are available than ever.

Respiratory Diseases

Illnesses and disorders like asthma, bronchitis, pneumonia, chronic obstructive pulmonary disease (COPD), and cystic fibrosis cause breathing difficulties and chest pain. They can put a strain on the heart and muscles due to a lack of oxygen. They are usually treated with medication.

Diabetes

There are two types of diabetes. The most common, Type 2, is characterized by the body being unable to produce enough insulin, while Type 1 is a lifelong condition in which the immune system attacks insulin-producing cells. People that have Type 2 diabetes can reduce the risk and effects of it with medication and lifestyle changes like healthy eating and regular exercise. In contrast, Type 1 can only be treated with medication. Diabetes can cause high blood pressure, kidney disease, heart disease, and even sight loss.

Arthritis

Arthritis is a long-term condition, often occurring later in life (though not always), in which joints become swollen, stiff, and painful, making physical activity uncomfortable or difficult. It primarily affects the spine, knees, hips, and hands. There are many types of arthritis, including rheumatoid, osteoarthritis, gout, and fibromyalgia, so getting an accurate diagnosis is essential if you start to notice symptoms since each is treated differently. Treatments to reduce swelling can slow the progress of arthritis, while surgery and pain management are long-term options.

Osteoporosis

This condition weakens the bones causing them to become brittle and more likely to fracture and break. It can take years to develop and is often only diagnosed once a break has occurred, most often in the hips, spine, or wrists due to a fall. Osteoporosis is common in older people, and women are particularly prone to it after menopause. The only treatments are avoidance—avoiding breakages as much as possible—and taking bone-strengthening medication.

Obesity

Obesity, or carrying excessive body fat, is a serious medical condition with many associated health risks, including stroke, cancer, heart disease, and type 2 diabetes. It also negatively impacts mental health and quality of life. While over-eating foods with high-fat content are prime causes of obesity, there can also be medical and genetic reasons, such as an underactive thyroid gland or taking steroids. Obesity can be treated with regular exercise and a reduced-calorie diet, though medication or surgery may be necessary in some extreme cases.

Chronic pain

Chronic pain is persistent pain lasting for weeks or months, usually caused by an injury or operation, although it can also appear in times of increased stress or unhappiness. Sufferers can subside the pain with medication and applied heat, but physical therapy, lifestyle changes, exercise, and even psychotherapy can be very effective for long-term relief.

Neurological disorders

These are conditions that affect the nerves, brain, and spinal cord, caused by abnormalities in the nervous system. There are many different neurological disorders, including epilepsy and seizures, Alzheimer's disease and dementia, Parkinson's disease, and strokes. They are all complex conditions with specialized treatments and varying symptoms, though, for many, the risk grows with age. Genetic and environmental factors most often cause them, though injury, drug use, and brain infections can cause epilepsy and seizures too.

Infectious diseases

We've all had cold and flu at some point—often multiple times a year—but there are many infectious diseases out there that we are at risk of catching without warning, such as hepatitis, Lyme disease, measles, stomach flu, sexually transmitted infections, HIV/AIDS, and tuberculosis. These diseases can be caused by bacteria, fungi, parasites, viruses, or through direct contact transmission, food contamination, or bites. Symptoms can include prolonged fever, fatigue, coughing, diarrhea, and severe headaches, and it is best to get a doctor's diagnosis so you can receive the proper treatment. You can prevent most infectious diseases by getting vaccinations, preparing food safely, washing hands regularly, and practicing safe sex.

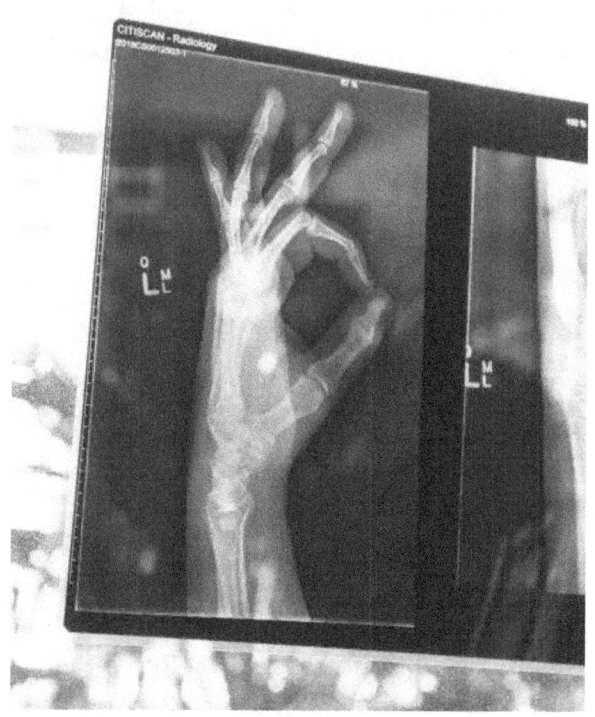

THE MENTAL AND PHYSICAL CONNECTION

Since mental and physical health are intrinsically linked, both significantly impact the other. The risk of developing a mental health problem is increased considerably by physical health problems, and vice versa. People suffering from physical health conditions may experience long-term pain and a loss of control over their body, which can lead to depression, anxiety, and low self-esteem, and those with serious health problems can also become isolated by their illnesses, unable to play an active part in society and maintain healthy relationships. When you are unable to exercise and socialize, you can quickly fall into negative thinking patterns and feel trapped, lonely, and hopeless. If your physical health increases fatigue, you are more likely to feel despondent and struggle to find the energy to socialize even more. Sometimes physical disorders lead to weight changes, skin conditions, and hair loss, which can have a negative impact on self-image. Being diagnosed with certain illnesses, particularly ones like cancer or HIV/AIDS, is enough to cause anxiety and stress and lead to depression.

Personal experience has proven to us how quickly one pillar can start to crack and weaken when the other pillar begins to crumble. Just this year, one of your authors experienced an injury that rapidly diminished their physical health, leading to a plummet in their mental health just as quickly. We have first-hand proof of how something as small and insignificant as a broken big toe can drastically impact your life. Excruciating pain, and a walking boot, meant no physical exercise or activities for several months. The first pillar breaks. This led to prompt weight gain that caused a tremendous negative impact on your author mentally. Depression and anxiety began to set in. The second pillar began to crumble. The injury took nearly seven months to heal (well enough) to resume a regular exercise routine, getting the author back to their original weight and improving their mental health. The physical health pillar was standing again, and the mental health pillar was starting to rebuild. We fully understand the power of the two pillars working in unison.

The brain plays one of the most vital roles in our bodies, so when our mental health suffers, it also directly impacts the body. If the brain cannot function healthily, neither can the body. Mental health problems can be linked to physical symptoms like headaches, fatigue, stomach and digestive issues, heart disease, and respiratory problems. They can also lead to insomnia and sleep apnea—which have a noticeably negative effect on the body—and difficulty concentrating, which can increase stress. Those suffering from mental health problems are also more likely to turn to smoking, drinking, and occasionally drugs to help them cope, and all of these come with severe and significant physical health impacts, including cancer, heart disease, and addiction. Adverse mental health has the ripple effect of making us feel less energized, so exercising routinely becomes a struggle, making us more likely to develop unhealthy eating habits leading to obesity or eating disorders.

Yet, for all these negative connections, there are many positive ones! The power of the mind over the body, and the other way around, can be used to combat disorders and improve health and quality of life. Exercise is proven to reduce stress and elevate our moods, so both mind and body are positively impacted, and maintaining a healthy and enjoyable diet nourishes your body and mind equally. These lifestyle choices put you in control of your health, reduce the risk of physical injury and illness, and keep you focused, centered, and energized. In later chapters, we'll closely explore factors like exercise and diet to increase understanding and awareness of the positive power of the two pillars of mental and physical health over our lives.

INTERACTIVE ELEMENT: HEALTH INVENTORY

Now you have a deeper understanding of the factors that are involved in mental and physical health and the critical connection between the two. It's time to start your journey toward taking control of your life and health and wielding the power of mind and body to your advantage. We'll start with a health inventory, so you can understand where you are starting from and form a clear idea of where you would like to end up.

Go to **https://bvhealthyliving.org/HealthInventory** to receive your free copy of the Interactive Health Inventory automatically, if you haven't done so already. These questions will help you assess your current physical and mental health and start to pinpoint areas that need attention and improvement. Answer them honestly and openly, without judgment or guilt, and know they are for you only to help you take the following steps to a better life.

Your Mental and Physical Health Inventory

To begin, answer these questions to get a baseline for your health:

- Do you currently have any physical health disorders?
- Do you currently have a diagnosed mental health disorder?
- Do any of your close relatives have:

  - A heart condition?
  - Respiratory problems?
  - Diabetes or weight-related problems?

- Is there a family history of:

  - Addiction?
  - Cancer?
  - Mental health disorders?

Based on your answers, you can already see some of the major factors that can have an impact on your health. When a family history of illness is involved, it is best to get a full physical from a doctor and discuss the potential dangers to your own health from genetic diseases and disorders.

Now, it's time for the questionnaire! Answer honestly and without overthinking to get the most accurate results. The questions are divided into three sections—mental, physical, and nutritional health. For each question, answer on a scale of 1-5:

- 1 = Always
- 2 = Frequently
- 3 = Sometimes
- 4 = Rarely
- 5 = Never

MENTAL HEALTH

1. I find it easy and fulfilling to discuss my problems with others.
2. I don't bottle up my feelings.
3. I don't feel stressed or anxious every day.
4. I make time for myself or my hobbies every day.
5. I meet up with my friends or family every week.
6. I practice self-care or self-reflection at least once a week (e.g., journaling, pampering, meditation).

PHYSICAL HEALTH

7. I do vigorous cardio-based exercise (e.g., swimming or running) at least three times a week.

8. I do stretching or strengthening exercises (e.g., yoga, Pilates, or weight lifting) at least three times a week.

9. I sleep 7-9 hours every night.

10. I make time for an exercise-related hobby (e.g., hiking) every week.

11. When I am injured or unwell, I seek medical help and advice.

12. I practice monthly self-examinations for cancer.

13. I have dental check-ups twice a year.

14. I maintain a healthy weight for my age/height/body type etc.

NUTRITION

15. I eat a varied diet from a wide range of food groups.

16. I avoid ultra-processed foods, which are high in fat and sugar.

17. I eat breakfast.

18. I don't snack between meals.

19. I limit my consumption of alcohol to the recommended amount or less.

20. I cook meals rather than order takeout at least
    six days a week.

Now, total up your score. Remember, whatever you score, it's not too late to make positive changes to your lifestyle and habits to improve your well-being.

- Less than 40: Great, you're on a good path to a healthy life!
- 41-60: You'll see some areas you can focus on improving.
- 61-80: Shows there are a number of areas that require your attention.
- 81-100: Indicates that you are struggling to lead a balanced and healthy life and need to make some significant changes.

Look at your answers and pay close attention to anything rated 4 or 5. These are the areas where you need to focus your efforts. Are there any patterns? Can you draw any lines between issues? Are the issues mainly mental or physical, or a fair mix of both? Did anything surprise you? Was there any area you've been overlooking?

Based on your answers to the questionnaire and the questions above, take your time to write down 3-5 goals for both mental and physical health to focus on throughout this book. You might want to prioritize your diet or exercise, or maybe you need to focus on your mental health—

whatever you need, make a clear goal for yourself. If you can, set separate diet, exercise, and self-care goals, as throughout the book, we will look at each of these areas in-depth and find ways to make positive changes using these factors.

Now you have a clear picture of your health and have set some goals to focus your efforts on. In the next chapter, we'll take a deep dive into nutrition, one of the crucial factors of a healthy and balanced life.

2

NOURISHING YOURSELF THE RIGHT WAY

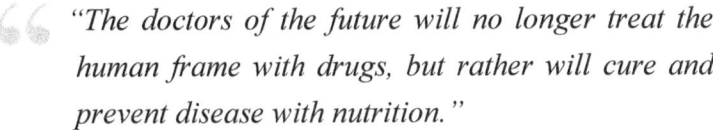 *"The doctors of the future will no longer treat the human frame with drugs, but rather will cure and prevent disease with nutrition."*

— THOMAS EDISON

Thomas Edison was spot on when he said that quote because food is perhaps the most excellent medicine of all. Aside from being delicious—which immediately ranks it high above powdery pills and nauseating syrups—it is natural and accessible to all, full of the goodness of nature and all the essential nutrition the human needs. A nutritious diet is proven to have incredible health benefits, from increased energy levels and clearer skin to significantly boosted immunity and organ performance and reduced risk of serious disease. So, what are you waiting for? It's time to set aside the sweet treats, salty snacks, and takeout and start filling your body with the fabulous fuel of a nutritious and delicious diet.

WHAT IS NUTRITION?

Nutrition focuses on the relationship between our bodies and the combination of nutrients we put into them. Nutrients are the essential vitamins, minerals, and substances required to nourish and support the body in its health, healing, development, reproduction, and growth, and we get almost all of them exclusively from our food, which is why a nutritious diet is so crucial to living a healthy life. Eating a diverse and nutritious diet helps you to stay fit and energetic, your organs and cells to function optimally, and your body to fight infection and illness. It also improves mood and helps to curb bad eating habits like binging and snacking. While you may try to eat a balanced diet, good nutrition can be impacted by lifestyle and financial factors, and time constraints. For example, busy people often turn to microwave meals or takeout to get the energy they need as fast as possible. Still, these meals usually end up needing more nutrients, and you have no control over the ingredients. Taking control of your diet and what you put into your body is the first step toward a healthier life, and it's a straightforward one once you understand what good nutrition entails.

The Essential Nutrients

A balanced diet consists of regularly consuming essential nutrients across a variety of foods. The body itself cannot make these nutrients in large enough quantities, so we have to get them through our diet. There are two different categories of nutrients; macronutrients and micronutrients.

Macronutrients

Protein, fat, and carbohydrates are all macronutrients. Macronutrients need to be eaten in large amounts and form the main components of your diet.

Protein is used for growth, healing, and strength; all your hormones and antibodies are made of protein. The body uses protein to make amino acids, which are vital for survival. Meat, fish, and eggs are high in protein, and, luckily for vegetarians and vegans, so are beans, nuts, soy, and some grains.

Carbohydrates are your primary energy source, fueling your brain and nervous system and boosting the immune system. 45-65% of your daily calories should come from carbohydrates. While low-carb diets have taken over the world, there's no reason to avoid them. Healthy carbohydrates like whole grain pasta and bread, high-fiber fruit and vegetables, and beans are an excellent alternative to refined grains, white bread, and foods with added sugar.

Fats are crucial for vital bodily functions like vitamin and mineral absorption, cell building, blood clotting, and muscle movement. While it is high in calories and often viewed as unhealthy, these calories are an essential source of energy and not to be drastically limited. Healthy, unsaturated fats are found in nuts, seeds, vegetable oils, and fish. These fats balance blood sugar—helping to prevent type 2 diabetes and heart disease—and reduce inflammation, lowering the risk of cancer and arthritis. It would be best to limit trans fats and animal-based saturated fats like butter, cheese, and red meat from your diet.

Micronutrients

Vitamins and minerals are the two branches of micronutrients. They both support the body's vital functions and are essential to a healthy diet and body. They are found in all food groups and are particularly rich in fruit, vegetables, nuts, and seeds.

Each of the 13 essential vitamins has an important part to play in the body and needs to be consumed regularly in the proper amounts for the body to function optimally. Many adults do not get enough vitamins, but they are easy to get if you eat a wide-ranging diet full of fruit and vegetables. Vitamins are antioxidants that are crucial for maintaining healthy skin, bones, and vision. They also boost the immune system, helping protect and heal the body, and they can lower the risk of some cancers.

Minerals, like iron, zinc, and calcium, are essential for many bodily functions, for example, hydration, strengthening bones and teeth, regulating metabolism and blood pressure, healing, and hormone creation.

Water

Water is crucial, and not only because it makes up over 60% of the human body. Water has many incredible effects on the body, acting as a shock absorber, lubricating joints, flushing out toxins, carrying nutrients through the body, hydrating, and promoting healthy digestion. It is also proven to improve brain function.

THE DANGERS OF DIET CULTURE

Diet culture has become a disturbingly prevalent part of society, with increasing pressure on people to aspire to certain body types, appearances, and lifestyles, often with an emphasis on food restriction, obsessive exercising, and avoiding "fatness" leading to overwhelming anxiety about failing to meet society's aesthetic and the consequences that will have on your life. Many of the diets and lifestyles we see on social media are unsuitable or attainable. Still, nevertheless, we try to adhere to them, often causing financial, physical, and emotional problems. Diet culture sets high, often impossible, standards for our bodies, and when you fail to attain or maintain the desired physical outcome, it can lead to shame, guilt, negative self-image, and a sense of failure. It also encourages negative, restrictive, and compulsive eating and exercising behaviors, which means things you should enjoy become punishing and unenjoyable.

Diet culture also skews our sense of worth, telling us that in order to be accepted and admired in society, you must meet specific physical standards regardless of your age, sex, body type, financial situation, and mental and physical health factors. It is essential to understand that health is not based on size or weight and that each of us has a different metabolism and body structure which means diet and exercise are different for everybody. An obsession with body image can have many negative impacts, including malnutrition and dehydration, constipation, mood swings, poor sleep quality, cardiovascular problems, muscle loss, and eating disorders.

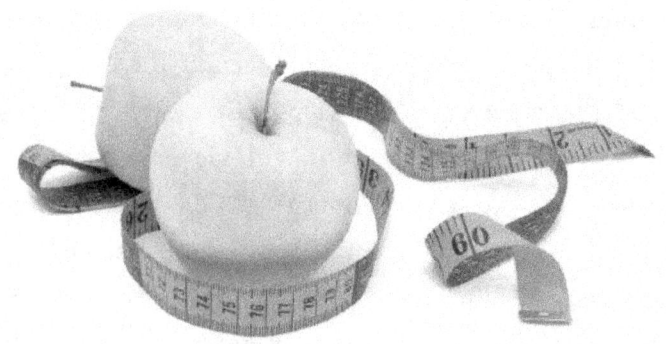

Symptoms of Disordered Eating

Eating disorders can appear gradually and be hard to spot, especially for the sufferer, so knowing the symptoms to look out for could be vital to helping yourself or someone else recognize when they are in danger. While eating disorders can be treated with mental and physical care, catching them as early as possible significantly increases the chances of recovery and decreases the long-term effects on the body and mind. Symptoms of disordered eating include:

- Preoccupation or obsession with weight, food, dieting, and calorie counting.
- Refusal to eat certain types of foods or food groups, especially carbohydrates and fats.
- Skipping meals or severely limiting portion sizes.
- Noticeable emaciation, especially gaunt cheeks and collarbones.
- Social withdrawal and avoiding social activities where food is present.
- Trips to the bathroom right after meals.
- Extreme concern about physical appearance— they may check mirrors constantly and seek positive reinforcement about their body.
- Changes or irregularities in the menstrual cycle.
- Difficulty concentrating and mood swings.
- Dizziness, fainting, and insomnia.

- Dental problems, including cavities, discoloration of teeth, and sensitive teeth.
- Poor immunity leads to slower wound healing and frequent illness.
- Dry skin and hair.
- Cuts and callouses on finger joints.
- Feeling cold all the time and blotching on the hands and feet.

By remembering that all our bodies are unique and have different needs, we can see the futility of diet culture. Instead, it is best to focus on building a healthy and nutritious diet and lifestyle based on moderation of food and understanding our bodies. For help with unhealthy eating habits, it is best to see a professional nutritionist or dietician and ignore social media entirely. After all, food should be delicious, enjoyable, satisfying, and nourishing, and should be allowed to be one of the great pleasures of our lives!

HOW DIET IMPACTS HEALTH

Physical Impact

The physical impacts of poor nutrition can be extreme and detrimental to normal bodily function. They can tremendously increase the risk of obesity, type 2 diabetes, heart disease, high blood pressure, cancer, and high cholesterol. With poor nutrition comes fatigue and poor brain function, including a lack of concentration and trouble with memory, and a noticeable loss of energy, stamina, and strength, making exercise more difficult and further aggravating the problem. The immune system is seriously impacted by poor nutrition, which causes frequent and more prolonged illnesses and difficulty healing wounds. Inflammation and oxidative stress increase, causing pain, anxiety, and even depression.

Mental Impact

A nourishing diet can also have repercussions on our mental health. Many foods promote a healthier mind, including green leafy vegetables, fatty fish, and berries. Nutrient-dense foods produce good gut bacteria that promote dopamine and serotonin production, which makes us feel happier. Foods that make us feel energized and focused, like whole grains and natural sugars, are remarkable for our mental health. In contrast, refined sugars and processed foods can cause inflammation, mood swings, and sugar crashes that negatively impact our brains. People struggling with mental health disorders are likely to have poor nutrition because they make unhealthy food choices that do not offer the body what it needs--they may skip meals, choose fast and easy options like takeout or frozen meals, or they may develop cravings or food obsessions that cause them to only eat one type of food for long periods of time. They may also turn to alcohol to boost their mood, which means adding toxins to their diet. Fatigue and insomnia caused by poor diet can also lead to mental health problems like depression and anxiety.

STEPS TO IMPROVING YOUR DIET

Over our 20 years of marriage, we have had our peaks and valleys regarding nutrition and health. Vanda came to the United States with her European approach to the pure and clean eating habits she was raised on. You can imagine the shock to her system when she met her fast-food-loving husband. She swiftly adapted to the American culture's quick and easy eating habits, and Marshmallow Fluff and Oreo cookies became her comfort food of choice. As we began to expand our family, we also started to expand our waste lines. Careers, college courses, and small children were the catalysts for quick dinner options made of processed foods and zero time for outdoor activities and physical exercise. We have endured our share of physical health problems over the years, such as high blood pressure, high cholesterol, sleep apnea, and vertigo. We came to the realization that we needed to make significant changes in our lives if we wanted to live a healthier, happier, and longer life with our family. It all started with improving our diet.

Improving your diet doesn't mean making sudden and extreme changes but introducing healthier eating habits over time—you're more likely to keep a healthy diet if it isn't restrictive or hyper-controlled. Building good eating and cooking habits is the best way to maintain a nutritious diet, and it can take a little extra effort. It is worth it for the long-term physical and psychological benefits. Here are some steps to improve your diet that you can enact immediately:

- Eat breakfast every morning! Breakfast is the most important meal of the day, jump-starting your body with a dose of energy and sustenance so you can feel alert and ready to work and your organs wake up and start functioning. Whole grain cereal or toast, oatmeal, yogurt, fruit, and eggs are all great breakfast options.
- Stay hydrated by drinking water throughout the day, not just when you feel thirsty. If it helps, set a water reminder on your phone to go off every hour or so.
- Eat at least five portions of fruit and vegetables. We've all been told this for years now, but it still stands! The fruit and vegetables can be fresh, frozen, or dried, and smoothies and juice count too, so there are many ways to meet this target easily. A fun way to incorporate more vegetables and exercise is to go for a walk and visit your local farmers market! Vanda loves to grow her own vegetables in her garden as well. Nothing is more

satisfying than the smell and taste of a fresh vegetable you grow yourself!

- One-third of your food should be starchy, high-energy carbohydrates like pasta, rice, potatoes, and bread—try to choose wholegrain options whenever possible.
- Aim to eat at least two portions of fish every week, one oily, like salmon or mackerel, and one meaty, like cod or haddock. Fresh or frozen are all great, though do be careful of smoked fish due to its high salt content.
- Limit your saturated fat and sugar intake. Saturated fat increases cholesterol, and sugar contributes to weight gain, strokes, cancers, and tooth decay and can cause erectile dysfunction! Packaged and processed food and drinks contain both of these, often in high quantities, so read labels carefully.
- Keep your salt intake to no more than six grams per day—a lot of our salt intake is in the food we buy, so check for low-salt options and avoid adding extra salt to food when cooking and eating.
- Avoid snacking between meals—if you get hungry, have some fruit or a protein bar, but nothing heavy or processed.
- Limit yourself to two caffeinated drinks daily and none after 6 p.m.

- Find ways to make your favorite meals healthier too. For example, use less oil for frying, swap meat for tofu or vegetables, or create your own sauces rather than store-bought ones. You can even make healthier pancakes with wholewheat flour and low-fat milk, and homemade pizza is easy to make and much more nutritious. We have had many fun family nights making homemade pizza with our children!

These are small but very effective changes you can make starting today. In the next section, we'll take a closer look at your eating habits and develop a plan to reach your nutrition goal.

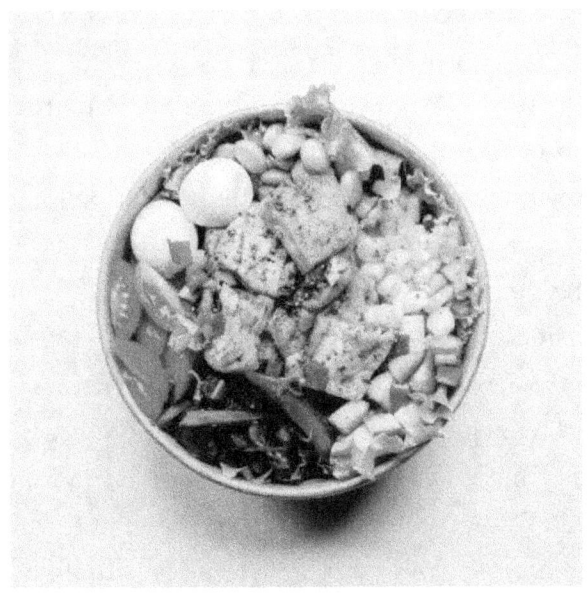

INTERACTIVE ELEMENT: EVALUATE YOUR EATING HABITS

Write down in your Health Inventory what you eat and drink on average each day of a typical week. Write down any snacks, drinks, meals, takeout, and any time you eat out, even if you get popcorn at the movie theatre. Take your time and be honest.

Now, looking at the list, look at it in terms of nutrition:

- Are all the food groups and essential nutrients represented?
- Are your meals balanced and full of vegetables?
- Can you count your five fruit and vegetables a day, every day?
- Are your snacks healthy?
- Do you cook from scratch more than you order in or have a frozen dinner?
- How much water do you drink in relation to caffeinated drinks and alcohol?
- Can you pinpoint any habits that could be considered diet culture habits?

Answer these questions by clearly identifying where your diet lacks nutrition. Remember, there is nothing to be ashamed of—you're on a path to improvement, and that's all that matters. From your answers, you should be able to see areas you can change your diet to make it more nutritious. Here are some easy ways you can make immediate and healthy changes to your eating habits:

- Write a daily meal plan for next week. From that plan, you can make a shopping list, pick up everything you need in advance, and be ready to start next week's nutrition journey! Meal plans are an excellent tool as they cut down on snacking and impulsive buying of food, and you know what you'll be eating, so you don't have to waste time and energy coming up with dinners every day. It also gives you control over your eating, ensuring you get what you need.
- Put a "no-buy" in place on the food you know is having a negative impact on your health. It can be for a couple of weeks or a month but stick with it and see how differently you feel afterward!
- Pay attention to portion sizes! People often overestimate how much food they actually need to eat in a meal. Food should leave you feeling energized, not stuffed. Weighing carbohydrates to ensure you get the recommended amount on your plate helps.
- Slow down when you eat! Try to take around 20 minutes to eat a main meal, and chew everything well. Also, try eating all your vegetables *first* to ensure you have room for them.

- Schedule meat-free days every week—just two days of vegetarian eating can make a massive difference to your energy levels and digestion.
- Try to eat a different dinner every day unless you're making use of leftovers—even then, spruce up those leftovers!
- Make simple but effective changes to your meals by swapping out bad for good! For example, swap fries for a baked potato or rice, white bread for wholegrain, deep-dish pizza for thin crust, chips for popcorn, sugary soda for sparkling water, and chocolate and sweets for dark chocolate, protein bars, or dried or fresh fruit. There are loads of great and easy swaps to make, so pick a few!

You can use your new knowledge of nutrition to work towards the fitness and health goal you set in the last chapter. The key to a healthy life is to commit to long-term changes rather than quick fixes, and the sooner you start, the better!

Now you're up to speed on nutrition and you've made positive changes to your diet, you'll soon feel more energized and in control of your body, so what better way to show it than to get your heart pounding and your muscles working? In the next chapter, we'll throw ourselves into exercise, one of the most important steps you can take to a stronger, healthier body and mind.

MOVING TOWARD HEALTH

"We cannot solve problems with the kind of thinking we employed when we came up with them."

— ALBERT EINSTEIN

T he first few weeks of a new exercise regime are notoriously tough on the body and mind, and the struggle can be disheartening when you are forced to confront the truth about your fitness level. However, if you can push on and commit, the long-term rewards are worth persevering for! The key is finding a suitable exercise for your body, lifestyle, and needs. While some people are happy to hit the gym, others find it an intimidating and pressured environment and prefer to work out solo in the comfort of their homes. Lifting weights and toning up work for some, while others prefer swimming or running to make them feel stronger. Everyone is different, and when it comes to exercise, recognizing that difference can help you form a healthy and productive relationship with fitness. It's *never* too early or late to start working towards a healthier and stronger body, and you deserve to enjoy the benefits of an active life.

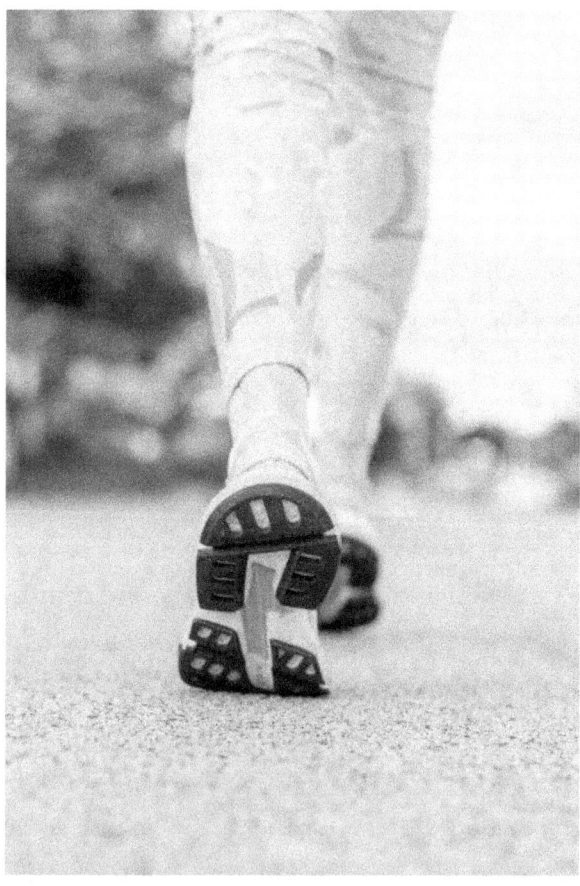

WHY DOES EXERCISE MATTER?

Exercise has a powerful effect on the body and mind—in fact, there are very few lifestyle choices that can make as significant, and as positive of an impact, as exercise! Engaging in regular physical activity is one of the best things you can do for your health, not only because it gets your heart pumping and your organs working but because of the numerous benefits it brings. Exercise is proven to strengthen bone and muscle, reduce disease risk, manage weight, and improve concentration, focus, and energy. Many adults find themselves in jobs or leisure time that involves extended periods of time sitting down, whether in an office or on your sofa, and all this sitting has a negative impact on the body. Notably, it can cause ergonomic issues that lead to weakened joints, bad—and painful—posture, weight gain, and fatigue. While you cannot change your working conditions, and while you should enjoy leisure time, you can choose to make time for some form of exercise every day, even if it is just taking a walk or stretching. Set an alarm to remind yourself to get up and move your body periodically during your day! There is a form of exercise for everyone, and everyone can experience the benefits of exercise, no matter their age, gender, lifestyle, ethnicity, genes, or size.

Most people's exercise journeys begin with a weight-loss goal, and while this is a commendable goal, it should not be the only reason to exercise! Even the fittest people, and those blessed with that elusive gene that means they never gain weight, should make room for exercise in their lives, and not just for aesthetic gain, but for their internal and mental health. Physically, regular exercise can reduce the risk of developing several cancers, type 2 diabetes, and cardiovascular diseases, and it can improve gut health, blood flow, and lung capacity. Although running and cardio exercises are popular, muscle-strengthening activities like weightlifting and yoga tone the body and protect the muscles from damage, while swimming, dancing, and Pilates are incredible full-body workouts. Finding exercises that work for you and your fitness goals and doing your research can also make a considerable impact—our bodies are all unique and need different attention, so if something works for someone else, be aware that it may not work for you, but something else always will!

The general rule is to aim to do at least 150 minutes of moderate physical activity every week. This can include walking, jogging, swimming, yoga or Pilates, or even dancing around the kitchen while dinner cooks, plus any number of other activities. One hundred fifty minutes sounds like a lot, right? It isn't! It works out to only 30 minutes five days a week, which really is a very manageable amount. You're probably thinking, "I have so much to do. Where will I find the time?" but it is infinitely worth carving out space in your day somehow, whether that means walking to work instead of driving, a morning jog, or a yoga session, a post-work swim (this is great, it really relaxes the body and settles the mind after a stressful day!), or a lunchtime walking session with your coworkers. Be the first to help inspire your team and build healthy habits together! As we'll discuss later in the chapter, there is always a way to incorporate exercise into your day, and even if you don't feel like doing it or you're tired, commit to it. Plug some of your favorite music into your ears that gets you going and inspired, and get your body moving! You'll discover you have more energy than you thought, and your body will thank you!

EXERCISE AND MENTAL HEALTH

If exercise works wonders for the body, that's nothing to what it can do for the mind! There is a magical quality to exercise. When you do it, your worries and cares fade away as your body takes over for a while, and your mind is free to relax and regroup. It's hard to worry about bills and the mortgage or get lost in dark thoughts when you're sweating your way through a Pilates session or counting reps at the gym. More than this, exercise causes the body to release "happy chemicals" like dopamine and serotonin that flood the body and noticeably boost your mood. Yet more beautiful effects are that it tires out your muscles so you sleep better and can wake more refreshed, and it increases your energy for the day by flooding the muscles (including the brain) with blood and oxygen. Also, exercise improves memory and thinking skills, contributing to an improved ability to handle stress. Partaking in exercise also removes the guilt of enjoying leisure time and food. In our modern society, productivity is the benchmark of success, so people often feel guilty for taking time out to rest and relax and instead find ways to mix leisure time with work time, for instance, by answering emails late into the night with only half an eye on the TV. If you've done exercise that day, you feel like you've accomplished something and find it easier to relax and enjoy food and time for yourself.

When it comes to mental disorders, exercise works its magic again. The increased sense of well-being it gives us reduces the symptoms of anxiety and depression and helps relieve symptoms of PTSD and trauma. In people with ADHD, it improves concentration and motivation. For people with eating disorders, exercise also improves self-esteem and gives you back control of your body. Exercise may not be able to cure these disorders, but it can go a long way to offering some much-needed relief from them.

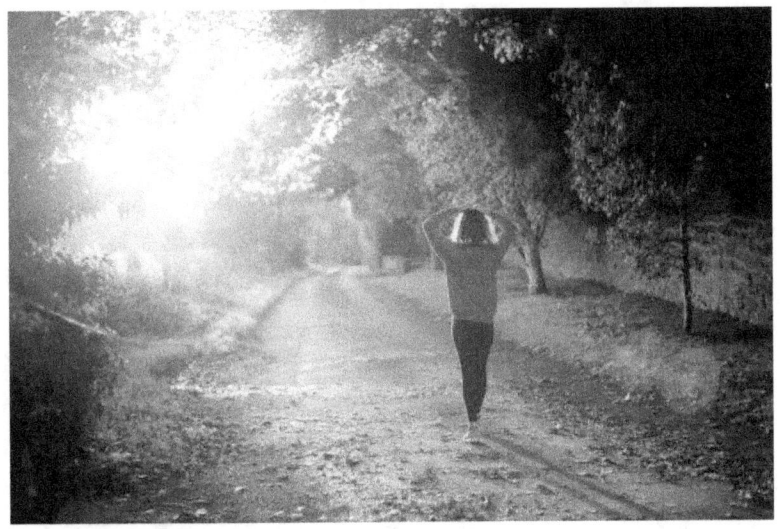

EXERCISING FOR BEGINNERS

Fitness Focus

Everyone's fitness journey starts somewhere, and the best way to start yours is by assessing your fitness level so you can make the right exercise choices and targets for yourself and your body's needs. Once you have a baseline, you can use it to measure your progress and see the incredible improvements you make in time.

Assess Your Fitness Level

You can assess your fitness level by yourself or ask someone to help you with the following activities. Remember not to judge yourself and simply do what you can—this is just the beginning of your journey, so you don't need to be perfect! Document your results in your Health Inventory checklist.

- Record your pulse rate before and after walking one mile (1.6 kilometers).
- Record how long it takes to walk 1 mile or run 1.5 miles (2.4 kilometers).
- Record how many push-ups you can do at a time.
- Record how far you can reach forward while seated on the floor with your legs outstretched in front of you—mark it on your leg with a pen to make measuring easier!
- Record your waist circumference.
- Record your body mass index (BMI).

Based on these results, you can set goals; for example, you may decide to shave 5 minutes off of your mile walk time within two weeks or improve your flexibility so you can touch your toes. Pick realistic goals and give yourself enough time to achieve them.

Design Your Fitness Program

Building your own fitness program is a great way to understand your body and goals, and also you can tailor it perfectly to suit your lifestyle, budget, and time constraints. Start by setting out your fitness goals clearly and realistically—remember that it takes time to build up fitness, so don't set goals and expect the achieve them in a week! Be honest with your abilities and the time available to you. You might have to move things around and prioritize, but keep your exercise consistent, as this will help it become part of your daily routine. Ensure that your exercise slots add up to 150 minutes of moderate exercise only or 75 minutes of intensive exercise a week, like HIIT training or dance classes—better yet, do a combination of both. Try to do some form of strength training for the whole body twice a week (yoga and Pilates are great if weights aren't your thing). Give yourself rest days; you'll need them!

Know Your Body

If you don't know where to start, your body will tell and show you where you need to focus your fitness efforts. Do you get out of breath quickly? Do your joints ache? Do you feel lethargic and struggle to get up in the morning? Do you have trouble lifting things? Does your dog drag you around the park more effortlessly than he used to? Take notice of your aches, pains, and physical limitations —these are the areas you should be working to improve.

Take a look at your body—not critically, not looking for flaws, but looking for areas you can tone, strengthen, and support. If you spend a lot of time at a desk, you might find your spine or shoulders are hunched, and your lower back is stiff. If you're on your feet all day, your knees and ankles may need strengthening. Find areas to work on but be kind to yourself!

Get Started!

The first steps of your exercise journey will seem like the toughest of all. Your body will ache, and your muscles will protest the new demands on them. You'll feel tired and unmotivated because progress will seem slow, but just start. The sooner you do, the sooner you can enjoy the benefits! Here are some tips for fitness beginners to help you through the first few difficult weeks:

- Start slow and low so you don't get overwhelmed, exhausted, intimidated, or worse, injured—little is better than none!
- Be sure to take the time to warm up and cool down before and after exercise—this helps to prevent injury and strain and makes the exercise itself easier.
- Be creative! Pick exercises that you enjoy or find inspiring, as you'll be more likely to stick with them. Combine nature and exercise if you can, such as hiking with friends.
- Be flexible. Not just physically, but with your time and plan. Unexpected things may throw it off, but don't let them derail the program. Instead, work around them and keep making time for exercise, even if it isn't what you planned for that day.
- Listen to your body.
- Ignore the mirror and the scale! You'll feel better in your body long before you see it, so it can be

disheartening if results aren't evident on the outside. Focus inwards and enjoy the feeling of change inside.

Monitor and Maintain

Monitor your progress by retaking the fitness test after six weeks, then six months, then a year (or as often as it makes you feel good), and you may notice you need to adjust your goals or routine. Health apps can be great for logging your exercise sessions so you can keep track of your active minutes and burned calories. If you notice you are struggling with the same exercise for a long time, or if your weight or size doesn't change steadily or at all, it is worth seeing if there is a medical reason for it.

FINDING TIME FOR FITNESS

In our busy world full of distractions, temptations, expectations, problems, and worries, it can seem like we already have so much on our plates that there's just no time for exercise. Our busy lives make us feel like we have to forgo fitness to face life's everyday challenges and errands, and when fitness starts to take a backseat, you pay the price. Here are some ways you can keep fitness in the foreground of your life and keep working towards your health goals.

- Capitalize on your commute. Consider running, walking, cycling, or jogging to work—or at least part of the way—if possible. Keep a change of clothes and some basic toiletries at work so you don't have to carry them with you.
- Keep workout clothes handy. By keeping workout clothes in your car or at the office at all times, you're equipped to switch into workout mode any time you have a spare 20 or 30 minutes.
- Run your errands—literally! Skip the car and walk, cycle, or run on your errands. This is a great way to get fresh air, exercise, and get everything done in one go, saving you time in the long run. If you must take a car to work or do errands, try parking as far away as possible to ensure you are at least gaining the most steps possible in your day.
- Schedule workouts as though they are meetings or appointments you can't miss—this will help you stick to them and prioritize them.
- Sweat while the kids are sweating! If your kids play sports or do activities, get a workout in while they're busy. You could run or walk around the field or park while they play or join in with them or the other parents.
- Get up earlier. Start your day just half an hour earlier to make time for exercise. This may be tough at first while your sleeping pattern adjusts, but a morning exercise session can help you feel

more energized and be more productive throughout the day.

- Find a gym close by. A conveniently placed gym that is quick and easy to get to will save you time on a busy day.
- Find a workout buddy! Working out with your partner or a friend can make exercise more enjoyable, social, and motivational, and you're less likely to skip a workout if it means letting someone else down.
- Keep a positive mindset. Don't let exercise become a chore that you just have to do—instead, find ways to keep it fun and exciting. Try new exercises and activities, get your friends or family involved whenever possible, and focus on the positives, like having more energy and a better relationship with your body when fitness gets tough.

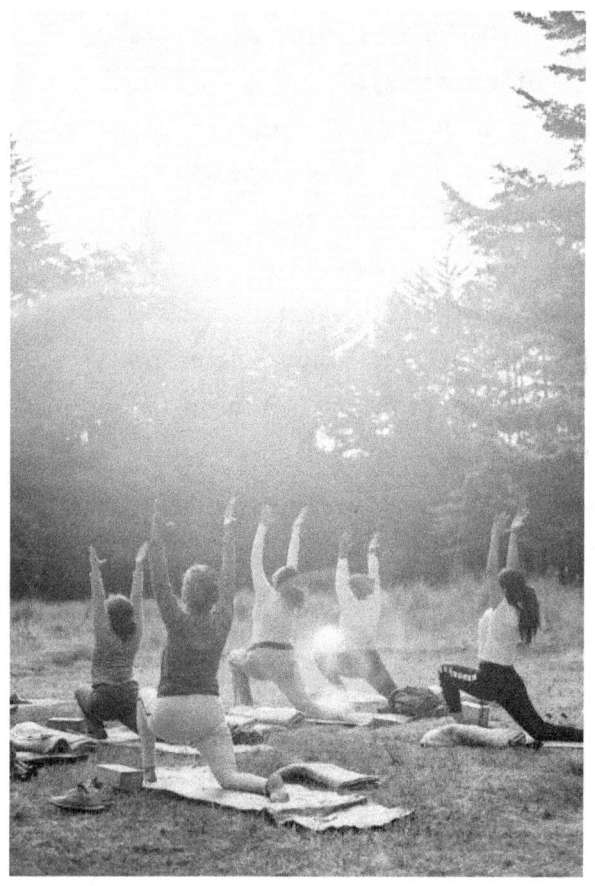

INTERACTIVE ELEMENT: EXERCISE CHART

In the Interactive Health Inventory, you will find an exercise chart like the one below, to help you log your fitness goals and progress and keep you on track to a fit and healthy you! Can you identify at least 3 opportunities throughout the day you can engage in exercise? There are opportunities even for the super busy individuals. Document a plan on the chart to stick to!

Finding Time for Fitness! Can you Exercise 3 times per day? (Target 150 min/moderate, or 75 min/intensive per week)	Results
6 AM • Are you able to wake up earlier? • Consider walking, running, jogging, cycling, or swimming to start your day more energized and be more productive throughout the day!	
7 AM • What can you try to implement? _____	___ Min Min
8 AM • Consider walking, running, jogging, or cycling to work. What a refreshing commute that can be! • What can you try to implement? _____	___ Min
9 AM • Get up from that desk and walk more throughout the day! Drink more water and stay hydrated!	Min
10 AM	Min
11 AM • What can you implement? _____	Min
12 PM • Can you go for a walk, or go to the gym on your lunch break? • What can you try to implement? _____	Min
1 PM	Min
2 PM • Get up from that desk and walk more throughout the day! Drink more water and stay hydrated!	Min
3 PM • What can you implement? _____	Min
4 PM	Min
5 PM • Consider walking, running, jogging, or cycling back home. What a refreshing commute that can be after a long day! • What can you try to implement? _____	Min
6 PM • Run your errands...literally? Skip the car and walk, run, or cycle to your errands! • Gym after work? Running, jogging, cycling, or swimming? Sweat while the kids are sweating? • What can you try to implement? _____	Min

4

A RESTFUL APPROACH

"A ruffled mind makes a restless pillow."

— CHARLOTTE BRONTË, ENGLISH NOVELIST

AND POET

Sleep is a crucial factor in our physical and mental well-being. In sleep, we rest our body and mind, heal, problem-solve, and reset, so we can wake up refreshed and energized for the day ahead. Those few magical hours of sleep are proven to have incredible effects on our mind and body, and you can definitely feel the difference in yourself and your energy levels after a good night's rest. It's ironic that in a busier and more demanding world than ever, we struggle more to sleep. We're exhausted by work and play, but our minds are so overstimulated by phones and so full of the anxieties of our lives that when our heads hit the pillow, sleep can often seem impossible. Night after night of disrupted or limited sleep, our worries and anxieties multiply further as our bodies protest and our minds become forgetful and easily distracted. Finding ways to encourage and ensure a good night's sleep is one of the most important steps you can take on your journey to a healthier body and mind.

THE SCIENCE OF SLEEP

In order to get a good night's sleep, you need to go through the four stages of sleep. Specific patterns in brain activity characterize each of these stages—these cycles and stages of sleep are known as sleep architecture. They are split into two categories: Rapid Eye Movement (REM) sleep and non-REM (NREM) sleep.

NREM Sleep

Three of the four stages of sleep fall into this category. **N1**, the first stage, comes when you have just fallen asleep. This short stage lasts only a few minutes, but it is easy to disrupt as the body is not fully relaxed, and the brain activity is still relatively high. **N2** follows; when the body temperature drops, the muscles relax, and breathing and heart rate start really slowing down. Then you get to **N3,** a deep sleep, when the body relaxes even further, and pulse and breath slow significantly. It is hard to wake someone from this stage of sleep. Now your body is in the perfect state to rest and recuperate—the muscles can heal, the blood can oxygenate gently, and all the physical strain of the day can melt away.

REM Sleep

With the body relaxed, the mind can let go too. REM sleep is the most crucial sleep stage for cognitive function—like memory, learning, and creativity—and for improved mental performance. In this stage, your brain dumps information, solves problems and experiences the most vivid dreams of the sleep cycle.

Are You Getting Enough Sleep?

Almost everyone will struggle to get enough sleep at some point in their life. It may be that you find it challenging to get to sleep in the first place, you frequently wake in the night, or you may struggle with a sleep disorder, like snoring or sleep apnea, that disrupts your breathing. Getting the recommended hours of sleep for your age group every night is essential to ensure your body and mind can function optimally the next day. Children require at least ten hours of sleep a night, while teenagers should get 8-10 hours. The recommended amount for adults is 7+ hours a night, and for people over 60, it is 7-9 hours. Of course, these are only guidelines, and you'll find your sleep hours vary depending on the season (in summer, it is light later and longer, so that can influence your body clock), temperature, day of the week, and your mental state—anxiety can play havoc with sleep! Let's examine the effect of sleep on our mental and physical health.

SLEEP AND HEALTH

Scientists are constantly conducting sleep studies to discover more about the vital link between sleep and health. Physically, sleep is your body's chance to turn all its energy to healing and recovery, which is why when we are ill or injured, we often feel drained, as our body needs sleep in order to nurture us. Relaxed muscles ease inflammation, pain, and injury, and in sleep, cells regenerate quicker.

The link between sleep and mental health is fascinating—sleep problems can be both a cause and effect of mental health problems, creating a vicious circle. A lack of REM sleep can impair the brain's ability to process emotional information and regulate mood, leading to an increased risk and progression of mental disorders. The fatigue and tension caused by an unhealthy sleep pattern can worsen anxiety and depression, and the prevalence of suicidal thoughts and behaviors is significantly increased by prolonged lack of sleep. Sleep disorders like Obstructive Sleep Apnea (OSA), in which pauses in breath reduce the body's oxygen levels, can disrupt sleep and are more common in people with psychiatric conditions. Insomnia is both a cause and consequence of many mental disorders, and the impact it has on our daily lives is incredible.

You are more prone to making mistakes, leading to anxiety and self-doubt; you may struggle to be creative, which can impact both your work and leisure; and you may feel enormous guilt and loneliness due to a lack of energy for social interaction. Essentially, while sleep won't cure mental health disorders, it goes a long way to helping keep them in check and reduce their negative impacts on your life.

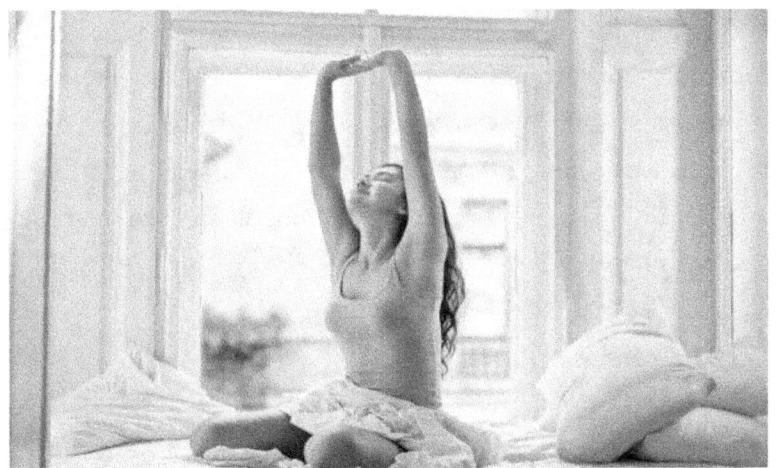

SLEEP HYGIENE

Sleep hygiene is the practice of keeping clean and healthy sleeping habits that help you to keep a positive and consistent sleep pattern and promote restful sleep. Good sleep hygiene is a simple yet effective way to improve your sleep quality dramatically. It helps you get to sleep faster, maintain sleep throughout the night and makes getting up in the morning easier. You'll feel more energized, focused, productive, and generally more positive in the morning. Building a stable sleep schedule is the principal aspect of sleep hygiene, as this gets your body into the routine of falling asleep quickly and like clockwork, rather than forcing it to stay awake or be unable to fall asleep when needed. Your sleep hygiene practices can be tailored to suit your lifestyle and needs, depending on your working hours, home and family situation, and any other time constraints. Whatever your circumstances, building a pre-bed routine and creating a sleeping environment that promotes quality deep sleep and reduces disruptions is the key to good sleep hygiene. In the next section, we'll look at ways to support yourself in getting a good night's sleep with some excellent sleep hygiene practices and habits.

Support Your Sleeping

You will need to change your environment and pre-sleep behavior in order to improve your sleep hygiene and sleep cycle. Making your bedroom the perfect place to sleep is a great way to begin.

Set the Scene for Sleep

Your bedroom should promote rest and relaxation, so start by keeping it clean and uncluttered—clutter can be distracting, and you want to avoid any mess that can cause odors and dust to build up. A fresh-smelling and clean room is not only healthier but also better for sleep. You can incorporate restful colors like blue, green, and orange into the decor, put dried lavender near the bed, burn relaxing scented candles or incense, and update your bed linen to sound quality, non-synthetic sheets that will allow air to flow and your skin to breathe. You can also spritz your pillows with a sleep mist and ensure you have a comfortable mattress and pillows.

The idea is to create a cool, calming, and cozy atmosphere. Your room should be quiet, dark, and not too warm—around 70-72°F is the optimal room temperature for restful sleep. Open a window to allow fresh air to circulate—you can close it if it is noisy outside, but have it open for a while—and you may also want to get thicker or darker curtains to help block out light and noise.

Positive Sleep Practices

An adequate sleep schedule is vital to getting your recommended hours of sleep, and these science-based sleep hygiene practices will help you to create the best conditions for gaining a restful night's sleep. Some of these practices are done right before bed, others throughout the day—give them a go and see how your sleep cycle changes!

- Develop a consistent sleep schedule by going to bed and waking up at the same time every day (allow yourself half an hour or so of leeway). This is one of the most complex parts of sleep hygiene for many people, as some like to indulge in sleeping in at weekends, and others want to stay up late watching movies after a long day at work. However, it is crucial to create a sleep schedule and stick to it, as this will set your body's internal clock and sleep drive on a regular pattern, meaning your body will know when it can expect rest and prepare for it.

- Build your pre-bed routine. Fill the hour before you go to sleep with relaxing activities like meditation, reading, taking a warm bath, or listening to music. Avoid anything that overstimulates your mind and body. Meditation can be a great way to let the day's worries go so you can go to sleep with a clear mind.

- Turn the lights down low. Soft, dim lighting at night is far better than bright, harsh light that stimulates our minds and keeps the body from winding down. Start setting the bedtime mood after dinner by dimming the lights and lowering the brightness on electronics.

- Unplug from electronics at least 30 minutes before bed. Phones, laptops, and TVs stimulate our minds and disrupt our body clocks, which negatively impacts sleep. Also, you may pick up a worrying work email or see a social media post that causes you anxiety and gives you something to stew over all night when you should be sleeping. Don't risk it—put the phone on "Do not disturb" or block notifications and leave the worries for the next day.

- Exercise regularly—but not before bed! Try to get your exercise in earlier in the day so that when evening comes, your brain and body aren't stimulated anymore and could do with sleep to restore them.
- Avoid food and drink with caffeine or lots of sugar at least six hours before your bedtime— they can stay in the system for a long time and disrupt your sleep. If you want a hot beverage, have an herbal tea like chamomile or peppermint.
- Avoid sleep-disrupting foods too! Acidic, spicy, fatty, and fried foods, and heavy meals, can disrupt your digestion and make for an uncomfortable night's sleep. You may get indigestion and heartburn as your body struggles to break down food when it should be resting. Try not to eat heavily within five hours of going to bed.
- Cut down on alcohol before bed. Alcohol interferes with the sleep cycle, leading to restlessness and shallow sleep depth, so don't drink any within two hours of going to bed.
- Stay hydrated. Have a glass of water before going to bed —but not too much—as this will prevent dehydration overnight, so you'll wake up with more energy. It can also help cool your body, and

if you have a cold or flu, a glass of hot water can relieve the symptoms, helping you get to sleep.

- Write a worry list. List things to do tomorrow or that are worrying you about the next day so they aren't on your mind when you're trying to sleep— they can wait!

- Use your bed for sleep and sex only. Avoid spending time in bed watching TV, eating, chatting, working, or social media scrolling—by keeping your bed for sleep and sex, you'll train your brain to see it as a place for rest and sleep only.

- Don't lie around waiting for sleep! If you haven't fallen asleep within 20 minutes of turning off the lights, get up and go to another room and engage in a relaxing activity like reading, a warm shower, or listening to music until you feel sleepy again. This stops you from getting frustrated by not sleeping and resets your body and mind.

- Skip the nap! If you have trouble falling asleep and staying asleep at night, avoid napping during the day, no matter how tired you feel. While a nap will boost your mood and energy in the short term, it will disrupt your body clock and make it harder to sleep at bedtime.

Start implementing these practices into your routine and lifestyle a few at a time, and see how your sleep changes! With time and effort, you'll feel stronger, healthier, and more energized and develop a more positive mindset around sleep. The two pillars of your life will feel supported and strong, and you'll have taken back control of the night and your body's essential natural cycle.

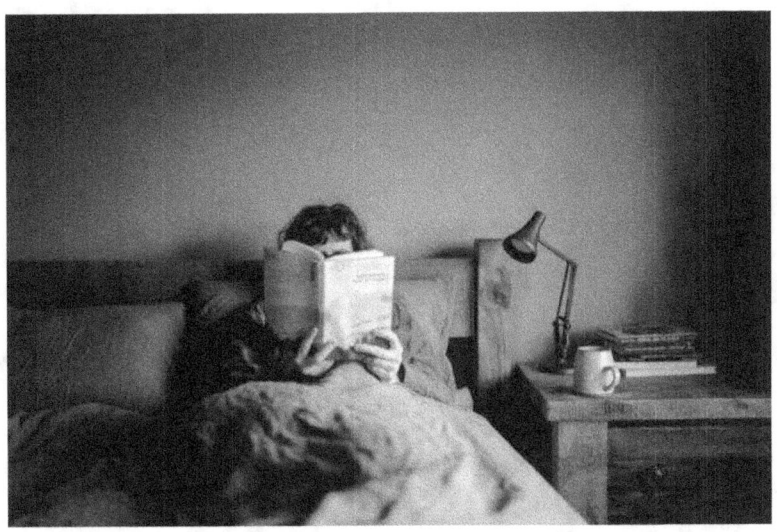

INTERACTIVE ELEMENT: SET YOUR SLEEP SCHEDULE

Let's start building your sleep schedule so you can begin your good sleep hygiene journey as soon as possible. Use this checklist in your Health Inventory to work your way through a nightly routine that promotes restful sleep and good bedtime habits.

- Have your final cup of caffeine six hours before bed.
- Have your dinner or final snack for the day at least four hours before bed.
- Dim the lights.
- Write your worry list—maybe with a soothing cup of chamomile.
- Open the bedroom window to let the fresh air in.
- Have a quick tidy-up in the bedroom.
- Have a warm bath or shower.
- Do your skincare routine and dress for bed with some calming music in the background.
- Set your alarm, turn off your phone—or at least the Wi-Fi—and unplug yourself from all electronics.
- Read, meditate, gently stretch, or listen to music or a soothing podcast until your bedtime.
- Drink a glass of water.
- Close the window if it is noisy or too cold.
- Get into bed and turn out the lights. Time to sleep!

The purpose of these good practices is to break the bad habits you may have gotten into that have been interfering with getting a good night's sleep. Bad habits creep up on us, and we often don't realize their negative impact until they are deeply ingrained in our routines. In the next chapter, we'll look at how to break them so you can retake control of your life.

5

SAYING "BYE" TO BAD HABITS

*"A habit cannot be tossed out the window; it must
be coaxed down the stairs a step at a time."*

— MARK TWAIN

W e've all got our bad habits, and try as we might
to ignore them or justify them; let's face it, we
know they're a problem! From little ones like endless
social media scrolling to the big ones that cause
emotional, physical, and mental issues for you and for
others, they all need addressing if you're going to
improve your life. Bad habits greatly impact our lives,
wasting our time, money, and energy, interfering with
productivity, encouraging toxic patterns, and preventing
us from living up to our potential. A vital part of taking
back control of your life is to break those bad habits once
and for all. You'll need all your patience, willpower, and

perseverance for this task, but you're not alone, and this chapter will guide you through understanding your bad habits, overcoming them, and building brilliant new ones.

DEFINING GOOD AND BAD HABITS

We have so many habits that we perform every single day that we don't even realize we have them. Habits are unconscious actions performed so many times that we do them effortlessly and without thinking, which is why we have such a problem identifying and breaking our bad habits. Since we aren't consciously controlling our actions but instead allowing our bodies to behave habitually, bad habits go unnoticed and unchecked. Bad habits can have detrimental effects on your physical, mental, and emotional health, including feelings of guilt, loss of sleep, heightened anxiety, poor eating patterns, and, in some cases, severe illness like cancer and heart disease.

Some bad habits are obvious, like smoking, drinking a lot of alcohol, or chewing your fingernails. In contrast, others are harder to identify because they form a small and routine part of our daily lives and can surely go unnoticed, but that doesn't make them worth ignoring. Some daily bad habits are far more noticeable for their impact on our lives, such as overspending, not exercising enough, and negative self-talk. These behaviors affect our bodies, minds, and budgets, and the short-term reward they give is not worth the long-term consequences of allowing them free rein over your life.

Some examples of everyday bad habits are:

- Poor money management, e.g., overspending, impulse buying, not saving
- Poor time management
- Not exercising
- Unhealthy eating
- Poor personal hygiene
- Slouching
- Scrolling endlessly on social media
- Checking your phone constantly
- Procrastinating
- Unhealthy sleep patterns
- Snacking every time you open the fridge
- Biting your nails
- Being late
- Lying
- People-pleasing
- Gossiping
- Staying in a toxic relationship or situation
- Overthinking

From this list, you might realize that sometimes a bad habit results from *inaction* or choosing *not* to do something that would be good for you, for example, exercising or eating healthily. Inaction is often the easiest option, requiring less commitment and effort than you might feel you can give at the moment. Because you're not actively choosing to indulge in a bad habit, you may not feel guilty or notice the negative impact of your behavior. Inaction is easier to explain away by making excuses such as being too tired or too busy, but these excuses are a sign that other bad habits are present in your life. As we'll see later in the chapter, actively working to change your bad habits is the only way to supercharge your life.

For all your bad habits, you're sure to have good ones too! Brushing your teeth properly, doing your skincare routine, and going to the gym are all good habits that you might already practice. Good habits, such as time management, healthy eating, and regular exercise, are the basis of a productive and positive routine that supports you in achieving your goals, keeping you healthy, boosting self-esteem, and reducing stress and anxiety. Good habits may take more effort to maintain, but the long-term results are incredible and life-changing.

Some examples of good habits to cultivate are:

- Good money management, e.g., budgeting, regularly saving
- Good time management
- Regular exercise
- Healthy eating
- Good personal hygiene
- Walking to the store rather than driving

- Maintaining a healthy sleep pattern
- Limiting TV and phone time
- Completing tasks in good time
- Being early
- Positive self-talk
- Self-reflection
- Saying "no"
- Removing yourself from toxic environments
- Giving people your full attention in conversation
- Setting boundaries

With good habits, the focus is on *action*. All the listed habits will take effort and perseverance, and you have to actively maintain and make time for them, but every single one positively affects your daily life.

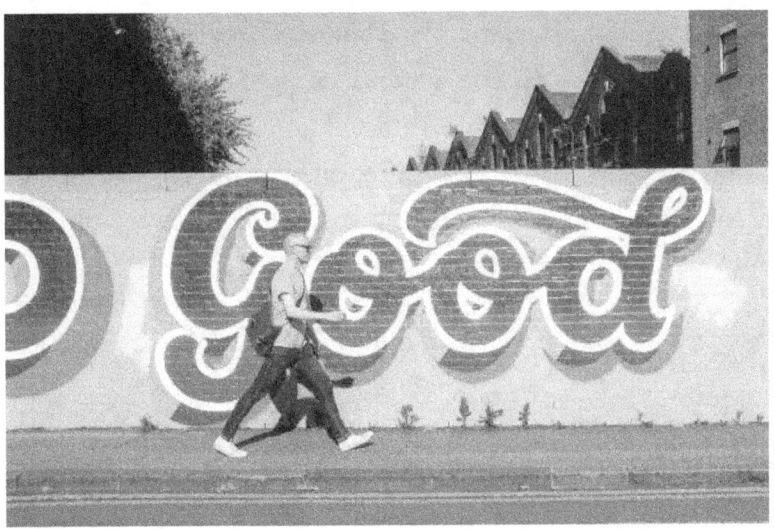

How Habits Are Formed

Bad habits form when the brain connects a **trigger**—like feeling anxious—with a **behavior**—having an alcoholic drink—and a **reward**—feeling more relaxed and less worried so you enjoy yourself more. Your brain quickly learns it can get short-term and immediate satisfaction from this behavior, and so it sends signals that cause you to repeat the action and behavior, chasing that feeling. Unfortunately, lousy habit behavior usually requires less energy and effort than good habit behavior, so bad habits often form far more effortlessly. There are other factors involved in creating bad habits too. Negative emotions, like those associated with certain mental disorders such as depression, can fuel bad habits, acting as cues for toxic and unhealthy behavior. Suppose you feel constantly depressed, anxious, or overwhelmed. In that case, you're more likely to pursue behaviors that bring immediate relief from these feelings rather than making positive life-style changes that require more energy and the rewards of which take longer to manifest, even though they would be more effective in helping you in the long term.

So, how do we break bad habits?

BREAKING BAD HABITS

Unsurprisingly, it is not half as easy to break bad habits as it is to form them, especially when they make us feel good or breaking them forces us to confront parts of our lives or ourselves that we would rather ignore. If you want to break bad habits, it's important not to feel ashamed or guilty about them but to approach them from a positive mindset that acknowledges them and why you need to change them. You have already improved your life from yesterday by choosing to break them today!

Breaking your bad habits will take commitment, perseverance, self-control, and self-reflection. That's a lot of energy and effort, so it's best to work on breaking only one or two bad habits at a time to avoid getting overwhelmed or burning out. It may seem as simple as just stopping doing something, but that can actually make you more likely to revert to your old behavior in a kind of withdrawal. Steadily working to remove the triggers and develop new routines to override the bad ones is far more effective and manageable.

Breaking Down Habit Breaking

Follow these steps for breaking bad habits:

1. **Identify your bad habit.** What behavior can you recognize is having a negative impact on your life?

Why do you want to change it? Understanding the effect it has on your life is an essential step to changing it. How will your life be better when you've broken the habit?

2. **Identify what triggers your bad habit.** Take a few days to track your bad habit and ask; when and where does it happen? Does it only occur in certain places or around certain people? Is it linked to another activity or event?

3. **Avoid or remove the trigger.** Change your behavioral pattern to remove the trigger and temptation. That might mean avoiding people, places, situations, or things that trigger you or simply not buying something, like cigarettes or sweets, anymore. Without the trigger, you will not activate the behavior.

4. **Replace the bad habit with a good one!** If it is hard to stop doing something, replacing it with something else—something better for you—can fill the gap, and in time, the urge to pursue the new habit will take over the old one.

There's a long road ahead of you, and along the way, there will be struggles, pitfalls, and setbacks that will threaten to derail your efforts, but try these tips for keeping on track to breaking that bad habit.

- **Start small and manageable.** Trying to break too many habits at once will be overwhelming, and you won't be able to give your full attention to them all. Instead, pick one or two that work together to break at a time.

- **Find ways to support yourself in your struggles.** It will be challenging at first, but you can help yourself by leaving reminders on sticky notes around the house, saying words of affirmation to yourself in the mirror, and putting up a list of the benefits of making the change so you can see it every day.

- **Find people to support you.** Family and friends can be beneficial as cheerleaders and goalkeepers for you. They can keep you on track to break your habit and may even want to join you in cracking the same habit for themselves! Some habits can seem impossible to break, but it is always a little easier with someone by your side.

- **Mentally prepare for setbacks and slip-ups.** Habits take a while to build up, so it makes sense they take even longer to break down, so don't expect it to happen overnight or without ups and downs. If you find yourself frustrated and falling back into old patterns, take a deep breath, identify where things went wrong, and see if there is a way to change your approach to breaking this bad habit that might be more effective. Most importantly, don't let doubt lead you to give up— remember that one bad day doesn't erase all your progress!

- **Reward your efforts and successes!** Keep yourself motivated to succeed with rewards and confidence boosts, and celebrate even small wins.
- **Don't be afraid to seek professional help.** Some bad habits, like addictions and compulsions, are tough to break on your own, and a mental health professional can be vital in overcoming them.
- **Change up your environment.** Walk a different route to avoid an expensive coffee shop, take the takeout menus down from the fridge, leave your journal on the coffee table, and avoid people and places that aren't supportive of you breaking your habit.
- **Filter out triggers.** Social media can be full of temptation and comparison, and it loves to show you things to distract you, so set filters to remove anything that might be a trigger or temptation from your feed.

There's no foolproof way to break a bad habit, but these tips should make the process easier and help keep you motivated and focused on your goal.

GROWING GOOD HABITS

Enough of the bad; now it's time for the good! When you replace bad habits with good ones, you open up your life to achieving your goals and potential. While bad habits make resisting temptation and negative behavior difficult, good habits flip that around and make resistance easier. It stops being a question of willpower and instead becomes a simple choice that requires no internal struggle—you just know what is right and what works best for you. Building healthy habits can seem like a mountainous and intimidating task—changing for the better constantly does—but breaking down the process into simple steps gives you more control and a more straightforward path.

1. **Set a specific goal for your good habit.** Be precise about what you'll do and when, and how often you'll do it. Doing a little towards your goal every day is a great way to make progress without overwhelming yourself.

2. **Plan the new habit into your routine with cues.** Cueing new behavior is a great way to make it a seamless part of your established routine, and it makes you less likely to forget to do it, for example, "Every day when I get home from work, I'll do twenty minutes of yoga in the living room before I make dinner." This is a firm and detailed plan and one that is more likely to stick and become a habit. The plan details the actions that will cue your behavior—in this case, returning home from work.

3. **Make it fun!** Find ways to make your new habit a fun and exciting part of your day; for instance, instead of just running on a treadmill—which can quickly grow dull even if it is effective—opt

instead for exercise that you enjoy and will look forward to doing, like a Zumba or Pilates class with a friend, or eat more fruit and vegetables by making flavor-packed smoothies.

4. **Be flexible.** In the early stages of changing habits, being strict can make the habit too difficult or rigid, so it doesn't fit into your lifestyle. Instead, have an ideal plan—like exercising every morning for half an hour—but be open to finding ways to fit it in elsewhere in your day. It might mean splitting it into two 15-minute sessions when you have time, but at least you'll do it! Being flexible makes it harder to throw off your plans, and it will keep you moving forward without frequent setbacks.

5. **Build a support network.** As with breaking bad habits, building good ones can be much easier with friends, family, and community to support your efforts, keep you motivated, and even join you on your quest. You could join a local running club, meal prep with your partner, or learn a language with a friend—there are so many options!

6. **Use reminders**, like Post-Its on the fridge or mirror or alarms and apps on your phone, to keep you focused on your good habit goal and to keep you from slipping back into bad habits. Your reminders could also be motivational, with

affirmations, commitments, or rewards written on them to help you maintain your efforts.

7. **Practice self-compassion.** Don't put too much pressure on yourself or engage in negative self-talk to shame yourself into action. Instead, stay focused on the positives of your habit journey, even when things are tough, and be gentle with yourself—remind yourself how far you've come and how hard you've worked, and tell yourself that you deserve the rewards you'll gain. Know that the only way to fail is to give up entirely and let setbacks fuel you to succeed.

Whatever your good habit goals are, there will be tough times, fun times, and with hard work and perseverance, success in the end. You already have everything you need to start today; willpower, intention, and self-belief. Harness your efforts and energy and pour them into making a better life for yourself! Think of habits as the ground beneath the two pillars of health. Bad habits make for uneven and unstable ground that cannot support the pillars of mental and physical health, so eventually, they fall, whereas good habits are robust and solid ground that keeps the pillars tall and supported, able to withstand the whirlwinds of life.

INTERACTIVE ELEMENT: BREAK A BAD HABIT!

For this final section of the chapter, let's create an action plan in your Health Inventory to break one of your bad habits and replace it with a good one. Starting small and working with the bad habit breakdown from earlier in the chapter, choose one bad habit that you know needs to change. For this example, let's try to stop using your phone before bed.

1. **Identify your bad habit.** Using your phone in bed before going to sleep.
2. **Identify what triggers your bad habit.** Perhaps it is boredom or feeling like you've missed out on something important happening in the world or your social group during the day.
3. **Avoid or remove the triggers.** Set app timers on all your social media apps to turn off an hour before bedtime. Turn your phone or the internet off before you start your bedtime routine. Put your phone on the other side of the room away from your bed. If you have a partner, ask them to do the same to help you with your goal.
4. **Replace the bad habit with a good one!** Have a book ready beside the bed and read for 30 minutes before turning off your light. Alternatively, you could listen to relaxing music or a guided bedtime meditation for 30 minutes.

Repeat this exercise for as many bad habits as you like, though try not to take on too much and overwhelm yourself with change. Start small, making little changes to your routine and behavior, and enjoy the big rewards of a life full of healthy habits! A favorite saying of ours that has become our mantra, small changes today make an immediate impact tomorrow!

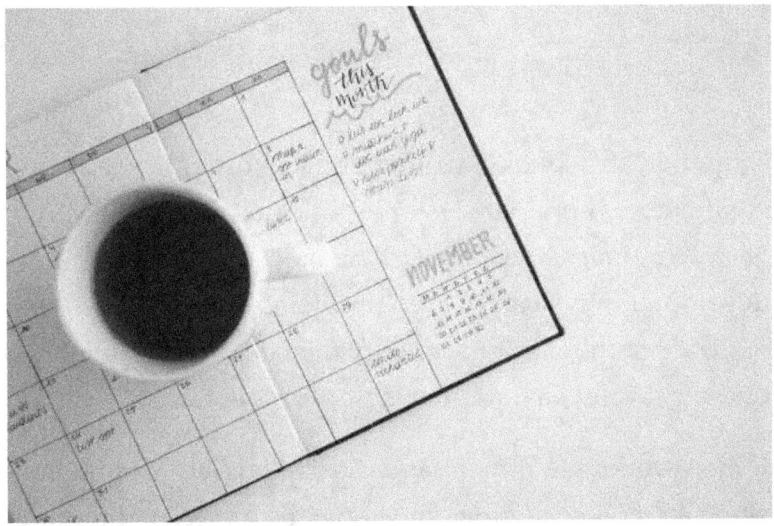

In the next chapter, we'll explore the power of self-awareness and its incredible impact on our mental and physical health.

SPREAD THE WORD: PHYSICAL AND MENTAL HEALTH GO HAND IN HAND – AND THEY CAN STRENGTHEN BOTH IN JUST 7 DAYS!

"True enjoyment is from the activity of the mind and exercise of the body; the two are ever united."

— WILHELM VON HUMBOLDT

Earlier in this book, we mentioned how quickly health challenges illuminate people on the inexorable link between their physical and mental health. They may develop a physical health problem, for instance, and realize that they lack the energy they need to socialize, go outdoors, or even complete daily tasks at home.

It also works the other way around. Anxiety and depression can be devastating, and someone experiencing these conditions can find it hard to maintain a job, stay active, or follow a healthy diet.

A myriad of studies have revealed that the link between the physical and mental cannot be ignored. For instance, one study published in *Nature Microbiology* reveals that there is a link between clinical depression and having low levels of specific gut bacteria. This is why so many experts recommend a fiber-rich diet—it can help you maintain good gut health!

Of course, working on your mental health by reducing stress, getting good sleep, and benefiting from the "feel-good hormones" released when you exercise, also improves your physical health.

Physical and mental health are two sides of the same coin. One cannot exist without the other. We are on a quest to ensure that everyone knows that they can make easy yet powerful changes that can revolutionize both. And we hope we can count on you to help us out.

We would appreciate it if you could leave a review of our book on Amazon, sharing your views on the mind-body connection.

Our hope is that someone who never makes time for themselves and tries to "soldier on" while neglecting their mind or body, understands two vital truths: they can make a change, and it is never too late to do so!

Give readers the motivation they need to develop a mindset that will inspire them to eat healthily, sleep well, and look forward to regular physical activity.

Scan the QR code for a quick review!

THE SELF-AWARE CHAMPION

> *"In our personal lives, if we do not develop our own self-awareness and become responsible for first creations, we empower other people and circumstances to shape our lives by default."*

— STEPHEN COVEY

We spend so much of our time absorbed in other people's lives and actions, living in on-screen worlds and working on autopilot, and receiving vast amounts of information that we barely have time to process before we scroll further and find more. This busy and wirelessly connected existence makes it easy to lose awareness of our place in the world, our actions, their consequences, and how we feel about things. We become disconnected from what matters most—who we are and what we really need to live a happy, healthy life. Without self-awareness, we become passive and unfocused. We lose sight of our goals and ambitions. We can lose sight of our morals and ethics and instead find ourselves fitting into the patterns and needs of others at our own expense. Rebuilding and connecting with your self-awareness is a vital part of taking back control of your life and living it on your terms.

WHAT IS SELF-AWARENESS?

Self-awareness is making the conscious choice to evaluate your thoughts, needs, and feelings objectively so that you make focused and informed decisions and take action for your own well-being and others. It is knowing who you are as an individual, how you feel about things, what you want and need, and being aware of your power and place in this world. People who demonstrate good self-awareness are able to connect with their thoughts, emotions, and ethics and know when their behavior doesn't align with them and their own standards.

There are many benefits to improving your self-awareness. It is proven to help you build stronger relationships, be more creative and confident, make better decisions, and communicate more effectively with others. Self-aware people are less likely to lie and cheat and more likely to reap the rewards for their hard work by getting promotions (especially in leadership roles) and other jobs that offer them the chance to progress and use their skills to their full potential. Self-awareness gives you clarity about who you are, and this allows you to pursue your ambitions with focus, understanding, and self-belief. It is a powerful thing to be sure of yourself in a confused and overstimulated world. It gives you the strength to stand firm in your beliefs and goals and not be swayed into acting against your own interests by the opinions, fears, or influence of the world around you.

States of Self-Awareness

There are two states of self-awareness, one public and the other private. Cultivating strength in both states is crucial to taking ownership of yourself and your life.

Public

Public self-awareness relates to our awareness of how other people perceive us. You get a burst of public self-awareness when you are placed at the center of attention, for example, when giving a presentation in a meeting or at your wedding. In these situations, you may feel pressured to adhere to what you think society and the people around you expect of you. You may change your behavior to "fit in," acting against your own beliefs and personality —you might laugh at jokes you don't find funny or pretend to agree with something that offends you. Often, people will experience self-consciousness or evaluation anxiety—worrying about what others think of them—in these situations. Notwithstanding, if you have a strong sense of self-awareness, you'll be able to brush off these worries and feel confident being yourself or presenting your ideas and opinions, even if they don't "fit in."

Private

Do you know that feeling when your stomach lurches when you see your work crush or realize you forgot to send an important email or pay a bill? That is private self-awareness. Our internal self-awareness is how we perceive and understand our emotions, passions, values, and aspirations, adapt and fit into our environment, behave and react, and impact others. By reflecting on these areas, we build a sense of who we are, an authentic self:

- We can more effectively make decisions based on logic and good sense.
- We can regulate and channel our emotions proactively.
- We can maintain control and focus under pressure.

The danger of self-awareness is that it can become self-conscious when you start to doubt yourself and your worth. This leads you to hide your true self and instead present a "socially acceptable" persona that isn't a true reflection of who you are—in short, people never get to know the real you. This can be a way of protecting yourself, but it also significantly impacts your ability to take control of your life and find success in your relationships and ambitions.

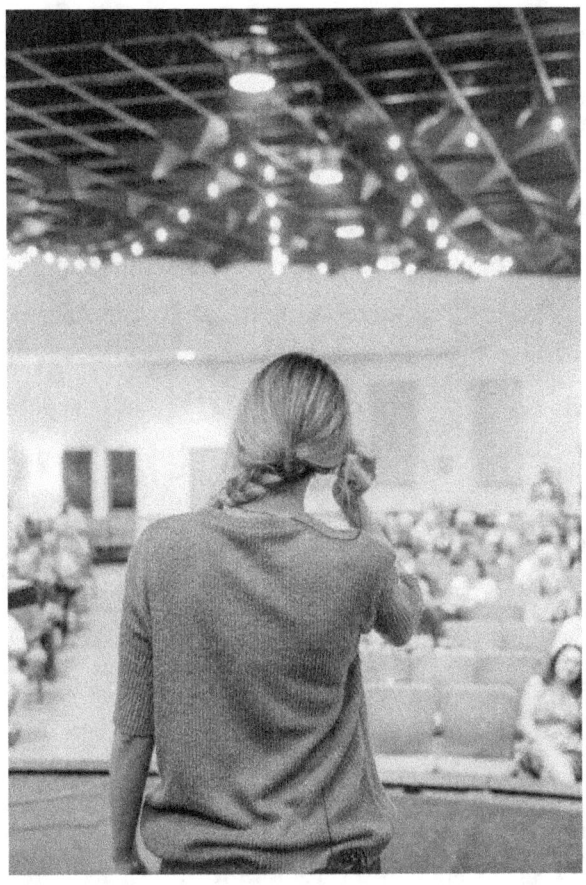

THE POWER OF SELF-AWARENESS ON THE PILLARS

Self-awareness can have a significant effect on our mental and physical health. With a healthy sense of self-awareness comes a healthy mind, which means a healthy body—everything is connected!

Mental

A lack of self-awareness can lead us to bottle up emotions. When those emotions are negative, it can lead to depression, anxiety, internalized anger, and resentment, which can then be turned outwardly as bullying or blaming others, leading to toxic relationships and loneliness or isolation. You could also end up people-pleasing at your own expense. Also, excessive self-consciousness can lead to social anxiety disorder, which can be debilitating. This shows how important it is to work to improve your self-awareness to benefit your mental health. Some of the significant benefits of a good sense of self-awareness are:

- Improved communication, which means you can express yourself and your needs more clearly.
- Builds empathy and understanding, promoting positive relationships.
- Improved self-confidence so we feel happier in ourselves and our appearance.

- Decreased stress since you are more assured of your ability to cope under pressure.
- Improved emotional intelligence (EQ): The ability to regulate your emotions so they don't rule you and express them in a healthy and productive way.

With private self-awareness and a healthy sense of self, you are more likely to have job and relationship satisfaction and a sense of control over your social, professional, and personal life, which leads to a happier and more stable mindset and a low likelihood of developing depression or anxiety.

Physical

The physical benefits of self-awareness on the body are directly linked to the mental benefits. Self-aware people work to improve themselves, which means they look after their bodies better, exercise regularly, participate in active pursuits, and find it easier to maintain healthy eating habits. The grand connection between gut health and mental health means that self-awareness can improve symptoms of IBS and aid digestion. The positive lifestyle that comes with good self-awareness comes with happiness, which floods your body with happy hormones that give you more energy and curb your cravings—and let's face it, happy, confident people just look better!

HOW TO DEVELOP YOUR SELF-AWARENESS

Developing self-awareness means opening yourself up to experiences, people, emotions, and reflections that encourage you to assess yourself and your actions. It can be very eye-opening and sometimes scary, but the point is to grow and improve, to understand yourself better. Here are some ways you can develop your self-awareness every day:

- Journaling is extremely helpful! Noting down what triggers positive feelings for you will help you pursue good people and experiences. Journaling also helps you to evaluate your feelings, process emotions and experiences, and be more mindful.
- Meditation is excellent for centering and focusing the mind so that you can dig deep into a feeling, problem, or thought within yourself, rather than being distracted by the external world. It can guide you to deeper understanding and new perspectives and help you to listen to your inner voice so you can form your own ideas. With meditation, you can also take the time to be present with just yourself and your emotions, without judgment or pressure.
- Ask for feedback and work to improve based on it. On a personal level, you could ask other people how they see you or ask a coworker or manager to

give you feedback on your performance. You may not like what you hear, but accepting feedback and working on it will help you develop understanding and awareness.

- Check in with yourself. Take a moment to pause and check in on where you are and what you are feeling. You can do this anytime, but it is advantageous in times of stress, panic, and high emotion.
- Be curious! Explore and experience as much as possible to develop opinions, skills, and confidence.
- Open yourself up and drop your defenses. Allow things to affect you, and don't avoid something on the chance you may get hurt.
- Keep learning! Building skills and discovering interests will reveal new things about you.
- Try to see things from other people's perspectives. When you are upset or angry with someone, remember they don't see things the way you do and are in a different situation. Approach them with empathy, ask them to explain their point of view, and be willing to hear their feedback and side of things.
- Look at your life and ask yourself, what am I learning and doing that serves me? What do I need, or need to do, to obtain what I want? Pursue the answer!

Self-awareness ensures you go through life with your eyes and mind open and with the confidence to be yourself everywhere you go. Self-awareness will equip you to tackle problems with understanding rather than emotion, and you'll be able to set and pursue your goals with clarity and purpose—something that we'll explore in the next chapter. Self-awareness is a solid core for the two pillars, a hidden support that keeps them and you standing firm against damaging external forces that try to keep you from reaching your full potential and harnessing control of your life.

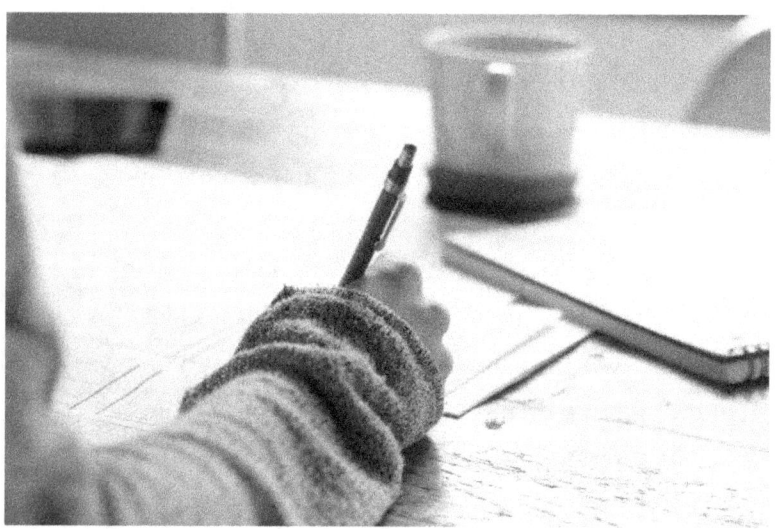

INTERACTIVE ELEMENT: THE SELF-AWARENESS WORKSHEET

Find a quiet and comfortable place to sit where you can focus. Grab your Interactive Health Inventory, a pen, and a cup of soothing tea. You will be working your way through a series of questions designed to enhance your self-awareness and encourage reflection. Answer honestly, taking your time to listen to your feelings and understand your desires. Allow this worksheet to take you on a tour of yourself and your life without judgment. Are you ready?

Breathe in… breath out…

Personality

1. What do you consider to be your best and worst traits/qualities?
2. What qualities do you wish you had?
3. What do you consider to be your five greatest strengths and weaknesses?
4. What do you like most about yourself?
5. What is one thing that you would change about yourself?
6. What song represents you?
7. What fictional character do you most identify with?

Values

8. What are the ten things that are most important to you?

9. How much time and energy do you devote to these things?

10. What do you believe is your most outstanding achievement?

11. What do you look for in a friend?

12. What are five things you like and five you dislike?

13. Who do you most admire in real life?

14. What fictional characters do you most admire?

15. What do you think someone would admire in you?

16. What do you fear?

Life and Goals

17. What is your idea of happiness?

18. What are three of your life goals?

19. What is a dream you have always had?

20. What is keeping you from achieving your dreams and goals?

21. What are you most proud of?

22. What talent would you most like to have?

23. Where would you love to visit?

24. What activities bring you the most joy?

25. What is your biggest regret?

Relationships

26. What is your idea of the perfect relationship with a friend, a romantic partner, and a family member?
27. Who can you be yourself around?
28. What has been the best moment of any relationship you have had? It doesn't have to be romantic!
29. What has been the most challenging moment?
30. What do you need most from a partner?
31. What do you offer a partner?

Appearance and Health

32. Do you respect your body and care for it?
33. What are your best physical attributes?
34. What outfit or item of clothing makes you feel happiest/best?
35. What is one area of your health you could improve?
36. When were/are you most content in your body?

Public

37. Do you always put others' needs ahead of your own?
38. Do you need approval from others?
39. What do you think people like most and least about you?
40. When you have done something wrong, do you ignore it and hope it goes away or try to fix it?
41. Do you avoid confrontation or speak up for yourself?

Based on your answers and reflections, identify areas you think self-awareness could improve your life, career, relationships, and health.

One final task. Can you remember a recent time when you lacked self-awareness? What impact did it have on you and others? How can you change your behavior and communication for next time? What can you do differently?

It's time to look outside of yourself now, at the world and life you have created, and decide if you're on the path to achieving your goals and dreams. In the next chapter, you'll learn how to set goals effectively and realistically to take control of your future.

MOVING THE GOAL POST

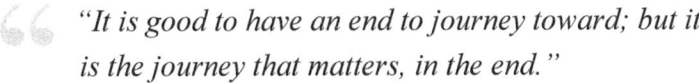 *"It is good to have an end to journey toward; but it is the journey that matters, in the end."*

— URSULA K. LE GUIN, *THE LEFT HAND OF DARKNESS*

Goals are an essential part of life. They give us purpose and direction, help us achieve significant milestones in our lives and careers, and give us a sense of fulfillment, achievement, and progress. With goals, we can gain sight of what we want and need in life, leading us to save resources and energy on less pivotal pursuits. We can strive for big goals that shape our lives, like buying a house, getting a promotion, or having a child. Yet just as vital, we must have small everyday goals that are stepping stones to those larger goals, like saving money and eating healthily.

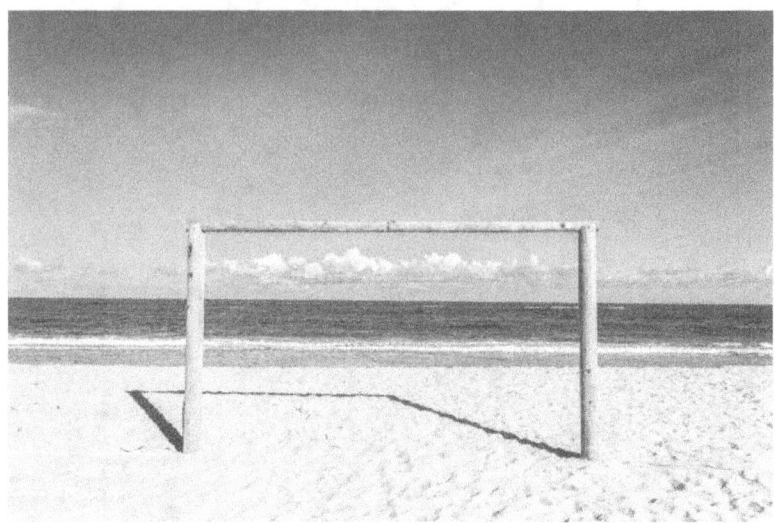

GOAL POWER

Goals are the destination at the end of the road, the roadmap of our lives. Sometimes the road is straight and easy, but more often, the road is full of hazards—hills to climb, cliffs to fall from, crossroads, and unexpected detours. Without goals, we would drift through life without purpose or direction, staying in places or situations that hold us back or hurt us, never taking risks or reaching for our desires. Our goals help us to prioritize our actions and understand what we value most in life, and they hold us accountable, even if we fail, forcing us to reflect on our actions and wants. They also help us to focus our efforts so that we don't waste our time, money, and energy on unimportant and unproductive ventures. Above all, they keep us motivated in the face of the many challenges of life, challenges that threaten to derail our goals and shuffle our priorities.

Goal Categories

You're probably juggling any number of goals in any number of areas all the time, and this is a good thing. It means you are aware of needing change in many areas of your life and are not limiting your progress. Juggling multiple goals can be overwhelming, so let's break it down and start by looking at the seven main categories of life goals:

1. **Health goals:** Losing weight, getting fit, going to the gym, and beating an illness are all common health goals.
2. **Professional goals:** These might include getting a promotion, changing careers, finding your dream job, and even leaving a toxic one.
3. **Educational goals:** You spend your whole life learning, so these goals don't stop with graduation! In adult life, they could be learning a new skill, seeking out knowledge on an area of interest, or taking a course at work.
4. **Financial goals:** In an expensive world, it is important to set financial goals, including saving money, budgeting, and paying off debts.

5. **Relationship goals:** Setting goals for your relationships is crucial to keeping them strong, healthy, and fulfilling for everyone.

6. **Personal growth goals:** These goals are aimed at becoming the best version of yourself, at making you feel good. They include making more time for things you enjoy or developing your personal style and appearance.

7. **Spiritual goals:** Goals for strengthening the spirit and bringing happiness into your life, such as volunteering, meditating, and practicing mindfulness.

It is usual to have long- and short-term goals in each of these areas simultaneously. Some may take priority or be more urgent than others, while some may require years of work to attain. Achieving goals in all areas is vital to living a healthy and fulfilling life and taking control of your life.

SETTING SMART GOALS

Whether your goals are short- or long-term, careful planning and clear goal-setting is the key to achieving them. SMART goals are a way of setting goals to make them as achievable and realistic as possible—they help give you clarity about your aims, keep your goals aligned with your values, and ensure your goals fit with your lifestyle and resources. So, what makes SMART goals smart?

SMART goals must be:

- Specific
- Measurable
- Achievable
- Relevant
- Time-bound

Specific

In order to make achievable goals, you need to make them specific. Making them specific helps avoid wasting time or effort on things that don't actually help you towards your goal. It breaks the goal down, making it more precise and less intimidating. It can also help you understand why the goal is paramount to you in the first place.

Answer these six questions to help make your goal specific:

1. **Who** is involved in achieving the goal/plan?
2. **What** goal do you want to achieve?
3. **Where** will your goal be pursued and completed?
4. **When** will you start the plan, and **when** will you attain the goal?
5. **Which** obstacles may hinder your progress and success?
6. **Why** do you want to accomplish this goal?

Measurable

By making your goals and progress measurable, SMART goals hold you accountable, help you track and define your progress, and keep you to your deadlines. Being able to measure your progress will keep you motivated, as even if you have a bad month, you'll still be able to see how far you've come in the months before.

Achievable

For your goal to be successful, it needs to be realistic, taking into consideration your skills and abilities, your resources, and any factors that could hinder you from achieving your goal. Your goal should offer the chance to challenge or develop your skills so you can progress towards it, but don't take on anything you don't have the time or resources for—this will only make achieving your goal harder!

Relevant

Keep your goals relevant to your lifestyle, ambitions, and needs, and stay in control of them. You might need support from other people at various stages, but keeping things in your hands as much as possible means you retain ownership of your success. When setting your goal, use these questions to make sure it is relevant:

- Does pursuing this goal seem worth the time and effort needed?
- Is now the right time to be pursuing this goal? Do you have other commitments or goals that take priority?
- Are you the right person to achieve this goal?
- Are you in a position to achieve it?

Time-bound

Setting a target date for achieving your goal makes you substantially more likely to achieve it! Deadlines keep you focused and accountable for how you use the time leading up to them, and you're less likely to procrastinate if you have a strict time frame. Have a realistic target date, but also consider what you can do in six months, six weeks, or even what you can do today to get one step closer to your goal. If your goal is long-term, think about giving yourself time to accomplish the short-term goals that contribute to it.

SMART TIP! Be careful not to set goals that rely on other people's efforts or that someone else has power over, for example, getting hired for your dream job. Ultimately, getting hired is up to the recruiter, not you, but your goal can be "Build the skills and experience I need to be a perfect candidate for the role," which *is* something you do have control over.

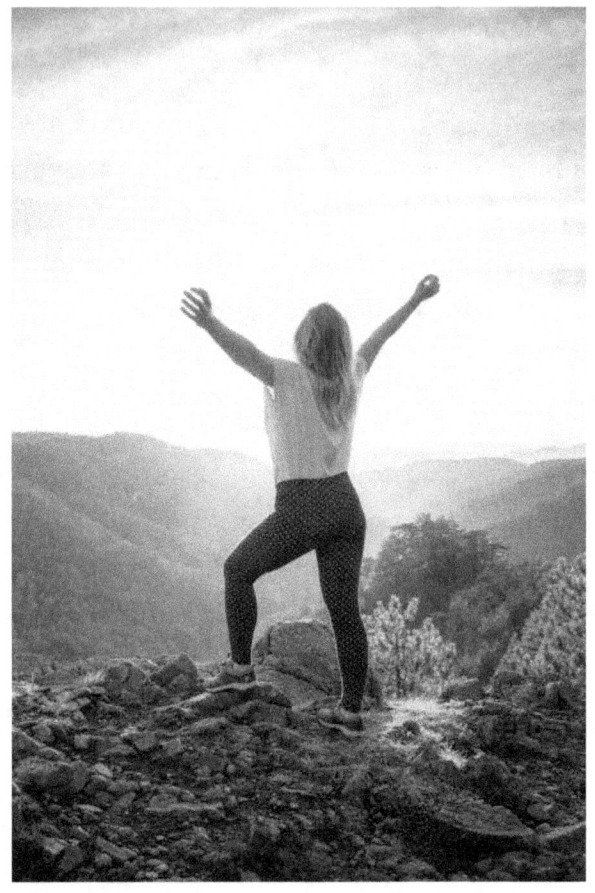

The Benefits of SMART Goals

SMART goals are a very effective tool for many reasons. They keep you motivated by setting a realistic and achievable time frame to work towards that allows for your lifestyle and any setbacks that might occur. This time frame also inspires action. Since you can't keep putting your goal off and waiting for "the right moment," you must get started and see it through. SMART goals also help to keep the end goal in focus throughout the journey, serving as a reminder that the hard work will be worth it in the end. The specificity of SMART goals helps you to plan the best way to achieve your goal in advance, making the journey to success as straightforward and achievable as possible. They encourage you to prioritize your goals and efforts, and they can help you identify why you may be struggling to achieve goals. They also can help you find ways to improve driving you towards success. SMART goals also force you to push the limits of your comfort zone by ensuring there's no room for excuses! By being time-bound, there's no room for procrastination and the comfort zone of putting off things you are worried about. Plus, you're more likely to achieve more of your goals and use your time wisely with the finish line in sight and getting closer every day!

Sadly, even with all these benefits and the higher chance of success, life's unexpected and unavoidable events can occur, and failure can still happen—so how do we deal with it and use it to fuel our efforts rather than ruin them?

MY GOAL FAILED... NOW WHAT?

For many people, the fear of failing is the main reason they don't set clear goals—it is easier to make excuses for failure if there is no plan to follow or deadline to meet—but failure is, unfortunately, a standard part of adult life. You'll never progress or achieve anything if you try to avoid it. Living with, and growing from, your failures is an essential skill to cultivate if you desire to live a happy and fulfilled life.

There are many reasons for failing to achieve a goal. Sometimes you work hard but don't quite get there, the universe seems to work against you, and the chances you were counting on don't materialize, you misjudge what you are able to give to the goal effort and fall short, or someone else gets there first. Everyone fails at some point, but the ones who will succeed are the ones who don't wallow in their misery and failure. Instead, they use it to fuel their energy to regroup, reassess, reflect, and move on positively and productively. Let's explore some ways you can use failure as a stepping-stone to success next time:

- Perform a post-mortem on your failure. Failure has signaled that there was something wrong with your goal, plan, or efforts, and if you ignore these signals, you'll only keep making the same mistakes. Doing a post-mortem is asking yourself, "Why did I fail?" and searching for understanding. It might be you overestimated your abilities or didn't work hard enough, you procrastinated too much, or you didn't give yourself enough time—don't place blame. Just identify and acknowledge where you went off track. Understanding why you fail will help you avoid those mistakes next time.

- Take a break and get away. If you feel too disheartened and anxious to try again immediately, give yourself space and time away from your goal before trying again. Taking a step back will help you see it with fresh eyes and give your brain time to refocus and work through the problem independently. Make sure you come back, though. Don't abandon your goal!
- Ask yourself the hard questions. Brutal honesty will help you identify where you went wrong, so ask yourself:

  o "Has what I've done justified this outcome?"
  o "Is this how people who have been successful in this area have done it?"
  o "If I continue doing things the way I am, will I achieve my goal?"

Use the answers to change your efforts and strategy to go after what you want!

- Seek feedback from someone successful in achieving this or a similar goal! How did they do it, and how did they overcome their problems pursuing it? Ask for advice, and act on it.
- Reflect on your progress and the positives instead of focusing solely on the negatives of failure. See how far you came towards achieving your goal,

and remember that experience and effort are
success too.

- Reevaluate your motivations. Maybe you failed
because you lost your steam or the goal needed to
realign with changes in your life or needs. Check-
in with yourself and assess whether the goal is still
what you want to pursue or if it needs to change a
bit to reflect new experiences, knowledge, or
other factors.
- Be kind to yourself. Self-empathy—not self-pity—
will help you to avoid blame and negative
thoughts that can lead to you abandoning your
goal entirely. Remember, you're only human, and
so is every successful person to do it before you—
if they can do it, so can you!

Your goals shape your life and future, guiding you
through difficult times and leading you toward the light of
success. The two pillars of your life, mental and physical
health, are instrumental in pursuing your goals.
Improving and maintaining good mental health will give
you the strength and clarity to know what you want and
focus on your goals. It will enable you to solidify your
self-belief, to know that you deserve to achieve your goals
as much as anybody else. Looking after your physical
health will give you a strong, energized body that can take
you on your adventures and bear the weight and challenges of your endeavors. Taking control of your life
means letting your failures inform your actions in a posi-

tive way that keeps you moving forward toward your dreams and desires, leading you to the life you've always wanted.

INTERACTIVE ELEMENT: SET A SMART GOAL!

Let's start taking control right now! Based on your goals from chapter one, choose something to develop into a SMART goal, one step at a time. We'll use the goal of getting promoted at work as an example. Grab a pen and your Interactive Health Inventory and take your time to work through each step of the SMART process.

1. Make your goal **SPECIFIC**:

   a. Who is involved in achieving the goal/plan? E.g., me and my superiors who will interview me.
   b. What goal do you want to achieve? E.g., be promoted to head of the department.
   c. Where will your goal be pursued and completed? E.g., My workplace.
   d. When will you start the plan, and when will you achieve the goal? E.g., I will start now by taking courses to increase my skillset, then apply for promotion in two years.
   e. Which obstacles may hinder your progress and success? E.g., How much of my spare time I can give to taking courses to advance my skills and experience and whether I interview well.

f. Why do you want to achieve this goal? E.g., I want to advance in my career, lead the team, and enjoy the pay rise!

With these answers in mind, write your goal clearly: "I will develop the skills and experience to demonstrate my ability to be the head of the department in my organization."

1. How will you **MEASURE** your goal? What will be the milestones that show you are making progress? For example: "Complete the necessary courses for the promotion and ask for performance feedback from a supervisor."

2. How can you make your goal **ACHIEVABLE**? What skills, abilities, and resources do you have or need to achieve your goal? What may hinder your progress that you can prepare for now? For example: "I will need to complete a course in... and... in order to meet the promotion requirements. I need to spend an hour every day studying the course materials."

3. Is your goal **RELEVANT** to your life right now?

4. Give yourself **TIME**. You need a clear and reasonable time frame for success. For example: "I will apply for promotion in two years and complete one course every six months."

This process can take time and research but work through each stage carefully to ensure you are building an achievable and motivating plan for your goal. When you've done one, try doing another!

Setting your goals is a great start, but you need to make room for them in your daily life to progress toward them. One way to make room for attaining your goals and removing unnecessary anxiety from your life, is decluttering and clearing out chaos in your home. Keeping a healthy and clean home is vital to maintaining control and direction in life, and in the next chapter, we'll discuss putting together an action plan to clean and declutter your home.

KEEPING A HEALTHY HOME

" *"Healthy people are those who live in healthy homes on a healthy diet."*

— IVAN ILLICH

Your home is your haven. It is your safe place where you can relax, unwind, and enjoy entertaining friends and family. You should be able to come home from work to a clean, tidy, tranquil, and welcoming home that helps ease the day's burdens. It should inspire peace and positivity, but it is easy to let negativity in, and once it is in, it can be hard to get it out. When this happens, the home becomes just another realm of anxiety and unproductivity, and a cycle of toxic home habits quickly begins as the clutter takes over and the effort to clean and tidy becomes increasingly overwhelming and impossible. This chapter will help you reclaim your home and make it a sanctuary for your mind and body.

YOUR HOME AND YOUR HEALTH

When your mental and physical health is anguishing, your home inevitably does as well, becoming messier and more cluttered as you add to the pile of clothes on the chair, dirty dishes in the sink, or papers on the coffee table. When you're physically and mentally exhausted, and as anxieties, illnesses, and obligations increase, your energy levels decrease, and you add onto the piles until your home is full of seemingly unconquerable mountains of clutter. At this point, throwing in the towel and letting your house be taken over is effortless, but that is the *worst* thing you can do for your health. There are many benefits for the mind and body in taking back control of your home, so let's explore them and get motivated!

Benefits for the Body

While the outside world may seem treacherous and unclean, your home can be just as unsafe, and since you spend such a large part of every day in your home, you can undoubtedly put your health in danger if you do not keep it clean. A dirty home encourages pests, mold, dust, and allergies, which all cause health problems. Bacteria spread rapidly in a dirty environment, and pests carry viruses, so offering them the perfect habitat to explore and make their home is a surefire way to get sick. Regularly wiping down surfaces, door handles, and food preparation and storage areas can make your home far safer in just a few minutes.

An unclean kitchen is hazardous. Bacteria and flies will riot if you leave dirty dishes, soiled tea towels, and basins full of used water lying around. You're also more prone to food poisoning from cross contamination and bacteria if your appliances, fridge, and cooking utensils aren't kept clean. Mold and dampness can cause lung problems if left untreated, so it's best to deal with them as soon as you spot them. Keep your home airy and uncluttered to stop mold and dampness from growing, spreading, and hiding.

On a slightly slapstick note, a cluttered house is a mine-field of things to trip over! You can hurt yourself easily by slipping on a greasy or wet floor or by tripping over a mess and clutter left lying around. Save yourself the bumps, bruises, and even breaks, by keeping the floors clean and clear of debris and wiping up any spills as soon as you make them.

Cleaning is also a great form of exercise. You can really work up a sweat doing a deep clean or even just a vacuum, and if you put music on and dance while you do it, it's even more fun and effective! If you're unable to leave the house or exercise at home, cleaning is a superb way to get your blood moving and your muscles working.

Studies have shown that you sleep better in a decluttered room too. You can relax and unwind much more effectively in a room where you aren't looking at piles of unfolded laundry or an errant sock that you know you should pick up but you just got comfy. A tidy room also allows clean air to circulate better, and clean bedding will keep bed bugs and other pests away. Better sleep makes for a healthier and more energized body!

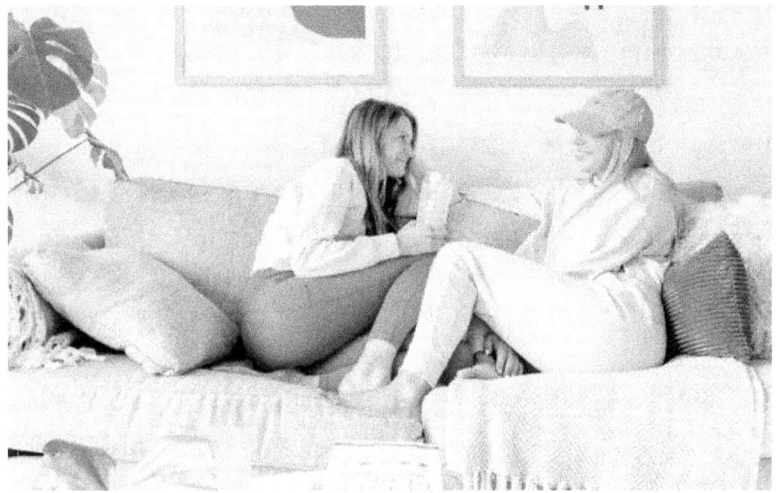

Benefits for the Mind

Your environment has a significant impact on your mind. Stressful, high-pressure environments make you stressed and anxious, while tranquil settings make you feel relaxed and safe—your home should be the latter. Keeping your home clean and tidy makes it a less stressful and more calming environment, and one you won't feel like you have to spend hours cleaning on the weekend when you'd rather be doing anything else. Also, a tidy house will save you time looking for things because everything will be where it should be.

A messy home or workplace can considerably impact concentration, creating mental clutter to match the physical. It draws your focus and distracts your attention, which can cause you to procrastinate and forget things. Keeping your home clear of clutter will help you concentrate and make doing the chores easier since you won't have to keep picking up and moving things to clean underneath them. Tidiness also helps to avoid overstimulation. You already have so much drawing your attention —phones, computers, TVs, social media—that it's nice to have a space clear of distractions and stimulations that you can decompress and focus on yourself in.

Putting care and attention into your surroundings is a form of self-care and self-love—you are showing yourself that you *deserve* peace and gifting yourself health and happiness at home. The mood-boosting energy of a tidy home is fantastic, not to mention decluttering and cleaning gives you a sense of achievement, so even on an adverse or unproductive day, you can feel you have accomplished something just by tidying a room. This feeling of accomplishment boosts happiness and self-image. Maintaining a healthy home also allows you a sense of control over at least one area of your life. Feeling powerless and unfocused is terrible for mental health, but exerting your will by managing your home can be a great way to feel capable, productive, and in control.

It might seem strange, but cleaning and tidying can be a very efficient form of meditation, especially for anyone who finds it challenging to sit and self-reflect in silence for a long time. Instead, you can keep your hands busy clearing the physical clutter and allow your brain to take a needed break from the mental chaos, giving you precious time and headspace to escape your anxieties and be present in the moment.

Finally, you're more likely to invite people into your home to socialize if your home is welcoming and clean, so you'll be able to spend more time with your friends and avoid the stress of a last-minute, frantic tidy-up when someone announces they are dropping by. Feelings of isolation and loneliness are damaging to mental health and often increased by a sense of shame or guilt about the appearance of your home, but keeping on top of your cleaning routine will free you up to opening your doors to the world and strengthening your relationships.

MAKE YOUR HOME A SANCTUARY

Refreshing your home and banishing the mess and clutter may seem an overwhelming task, especially if it has been a while since you tried or you just haven't had the time or energy, so let's break down the process into smaller steps to take back your space and make your home a peaceful paradise again.

Declutter

The first step to finding sanctuary is to eliminate the clutter and chaos that is filling the space with negative energy and making the task seem impossible. Decluttering is more than just tidying up—it is about removing objects and debris that cause anxiety and bring no joy to your home. Often clutter takes the form of hoarded possessions like clothes, electronics, and decorations, which get tossed about and overload the cabinets and surfaces so you can't find the stuff you need or want. Decluttering your house will show you the things that matter, make your life better, help you to bring order to your home, and improve the quality of your life. Here are some tips for decluttering to make it a straightforward and productive process:

- Before you start, ensure you have plenty of boxes and trash bags ready. As you declutter, segregate things to keep and donate into separate boxes. Only throw away broken items or anything too dirty to save.
- Pick **one** area of the house to start in, not a whole room, just a corner or a cabinet. Starting small makes the task less intimidating and helps to focus your efforts and avoid distractions. You can work

your way around the room and the house, area by area, for as long as you like—it could take one day or over a week. Just be sure to go at your own pace.

- Sort through objects individually, deciding whether to keep, donate, or throw them away. Only keep things that make you feel happy, are essential or valuable, and are used often.
- Have a microfiber cloth or cleaning wipes handy to wipe down surfaces and objects as you go.
- Donate unwanted items as soon as possible so they aren't hanging around the house.
- Use baskets, boxes, and wire zipties to make everything neat and keep surfaces clear.
- If you can't decide whether to keep or donate something, give yourself a deadline to use it, for example, three months. Let it go if you haven't used, worn, or needed it at the end of the three months.

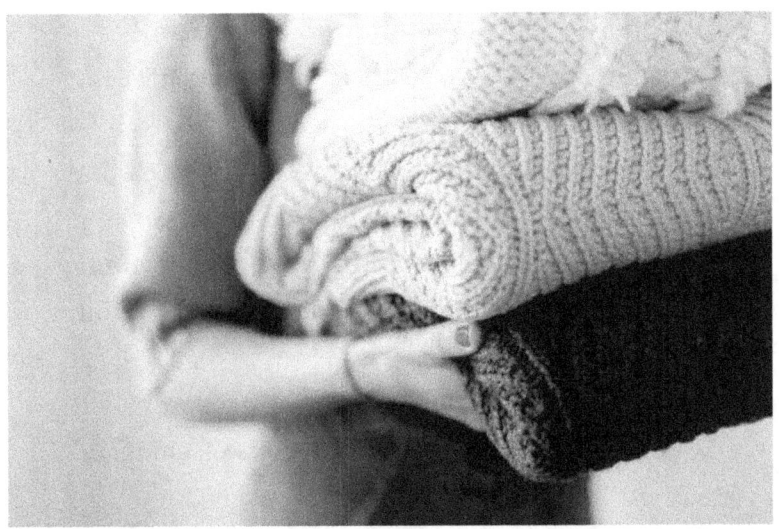

Conquer the Cleaning

It is easy to feel defeated, unmotivated, and overwhelmed in the face of such an arduous task as cleaning the house, so use these cleaning tips and tricks to take back control of your home's health and defeat the dirt.

- Set a timer for a realistic amount of time to clean —enough time that you can make progress but won't get overwhelmed. Get as much done as you can in that time. Even just ten minutes of cleaning one room a day can make a huge difference, and that ten minutes is effortless to slip into your daily routine, and it will fly by before you know it.
- Pick one area, or object to clean, and focus your energy on that. Sorting the laundry is a great example. Appliances like the refrigerator, oven,

and shower take more effort to clean than anything else, so make sure to give yourself plenty of time with them.

- Give each room a day of the week for its turn to be cleaned—this way, you'll be able to keep the rooms on a constant cleaning rotation that should keep dirt and mess from building up throughout the house.

- Use eco friendly plant based cleaning sprays, wipes, and microfiber cloths to make cleaning easier.

- Put on an energizing playlist as loud as you like to keep your spirits and energy up while you clean!

- Prioritize the cleaning tasks that have a positive and noticeable effect on the space, for example, changing your bed sheets or cleaning the oven. They will show you the rewards of your efforts and motivate you to keep going!

- Ask for help! Having someone to work through chores with you makes it more fun and the task more manageable.

- Make a thorough list of what to clean in every room and work your way through it—checking off your cleaning accomplishments will feel more rewarding and productive!

Decor and Design

How you decorate your home has an incredible and often overlooked impact on your health. There are lots of ways to improve your physical and, especially, your mental health with simple design and decor choices, such as:

- Fill up empty space with houseplants! They not only give out needed oxygen that improves air quality and aids concentration, but they are a fun project, and keeping them healthy and alive is very rewarding. Like humans, plants need love and care, so share a little with them, and they'll give it back.
- Use light and cool colors to energize and enlarge a room or warm and dark colors for cozy spaces.
- Don't rely on ceiling lights, which can be harsh and overstimulating, especially in the evening. Use lamps or fairy lights as night draws in, and candles can be very calming too—only don't forget to blow them out before bed!
- Fill your home with soothing scents! Scents like vanilla, lavender, rose, and cinnamon are remarkably calming and will make your home feel fresh and welcoming. Sage smudging is a great way to remove negative energy from your home too!

- Decorate to encourage joy! Bright colors and lively wall art can boost mood and energize your home.
- Choose blankets, duvet covers, and pillowcases in soft, breathable fabrics like cotton or linen to encourage cool and comfortable sleep.
- Keep to an aesthetic when decorating and choosing furniture. This will give your home a cohesive and controlled atmosphere which will help you focus and be more motivated to keep it tidy.
- Give yourself *space* to move and think. Encourage air and energy flow around the home, and don't fill the space with objects and furniture. Moving around should be easy, and less stuff means less to clean!

You don't need the stress of making considerable changes to your decor all at once, and you certainly don't need to rack up the cost of replacing all the furniture—take your time, work with what you've got, and add to your home at your own pace and within your budget.

INTERACTIVE ELEMENT: YOUR ROOM-BY-ROOM DEEP CLEAN CHECKLIST

Deep cleaning is an essential—and rewarding—task for maintaining a healthy home, but it can be intimidating and time-consuming at the same time. Luckily, staying on top of your weekly cleaning routine makes deep cleaning more manageable and less overwhelming. A deep clean aims to focus your energy on eliminating the dirt, dust, and grime that can get overlooked in your everyday cleaning efforts. You'll be cleaning the hard-to-reach areas that are typically missed quite easily and dusting and scrubbing the house from top to bottom. While some rooms, like the bathroom and kitchen, need a thorough wiping down every week, you'll only need to perform a deep clean on the whole house once or twice a year.

You will need:

- A mop and bucket
- Cleaning cloths—microfiber cloths are great!
- Multipurpose cleaner
- Rubber gloves
- A vacuum cleaner
- Toothbrush—for corners and drains, etc.
- Telescopic duster
- White vinegar
- Baking soda
- Window and glass cleaner

- Non-scratch scrubbing pads

Use the following checklist and the supplies above to deep clean every room in your home thoroughly, one at a time. You can break it down and do one room a month to make deep cleaning more manageable.

Bedroom

- Launder all the bedding, including the blanket/duvet and pillows, and wipe down the bed frame.
- Refresh your mattress. Sprinkle it all over with baking soda, leave it for an hour, then vacuum it thoroughly—this will eliminate odors. Don't forget to flip the mattress and do the other side!
- Declutter your closets and drawers, dust and wipe inside, and leave them open to breathe and dry well while you sort through your clothes.
- Dust, vacuum, and wipe down the baseboards and windowsills.
- Vacuum the curtains or blinds and clean the windows.

Kitchen

- Empty out your cabinets, and pantry shelves, and thoroughly wipe them down inside and all over the doors. While they dry and air out, go through the contents, throw away anything out of date, and wipe any residue off bottles and containers.
- Clear your counters of appliances, clean and dry them and the backsplash. Wipe down the appliances, and only put back what you use daily —find homes in cabinets and out of sight for everything you use less often.
- Deep clean your large appliances—fridge, freezer, stove, oven, and dishwasher—inside and out (you may need special cleaning supplies for the oven and dishwasher.) Pull them away from the wall to clean behind and beneath them if you can.
- Scrub and wipe down the sink.
- Sweep, then mop the floor with warm soapy water.

Bathroom

- Wash your shower curtain (check the cleaning label for which cycle to use.)
- Clean the soap scum and water spots from the shower doors and mirrors.
- Sort through the bathroom cabinets and clean the shelves.

- Use the toothbrush to scrub between the tiles, along the shower door tracks, and around the edge of the bath where mold and dirt build up.
- Mop the floor.

Living Room

- Remove and wash cushion covers and throw pillows, and vacuum the sofa and chairs thoroughly with the brush attachment for the vacuum cleaner. You can also run a lint roller over everything.
- Dust any photo frames and wipe the glass.
- Dust underneath any electronics.
- Dust the lampshades.
- Vacuum the curtains or blinds and wipe the windows and windowsills.
- Wipe the baseboards.
- Beat any rugs outside to remove loose dirt and dust, then vacuum the carpet and rugs thoroughly.

These tasks do not need to be done every week or even every month, but be sure to do them a few times a year, particularly in summer, when pollen, dust, and insects are everywhere. If you deep clean one room a month, you'll do them all three times a year!

Cleaning is one of the most important parts of your routine, not only for your health but also for your happiness. Routines, in general, give us structure and control, and in the next chapter, we'll look more closely at the ways routines impact and improve our lives and health.

A NEAT 7-DAY PACKAGE

66 *"The secret of change is to focus all your energy not on fighting the old but on building the new."*

— SOCRATES, PHILOSOPHER

As we have ventured our way through to the end of this book, we have stressed the importance of maintaining the strength and structure of your two pillars of power and stressed how vital they are to balance your life and happiness.

The pillars of your physical and mental health are indispensable to your power. Together they are the foundation of your entire being, and your life will be a difficult struggle without one or the other. The strength of both pillars is forged from the three main ingredients we covered in the preceding chapters. **Exercise. Nutrition.**

Sleep. Each piece plays such a vital role in building the strength of the pillars that they will begin to crack and crumble if one of them is unaccounted for.

Without proper exercise, your physical health diminishes, which can lead to anxiety and depression, therefore, affecting your mental health negatively. In turn, this can lead to poor eating habits and sleeping disorders.

Without proper nutrition, the body will not have the essential nutrients it needs to provide the energy required to exercise successfully and maintain a high level of physical health. Both pillars begin to crumble, and sleep is impacted yet once again.

Without proper sleep, you can abandon the thought of having optimal physical health and nutrition results. When you lack adequate sleep, you lack energy and are always tired and sluggish.

When you lack energy, you resist pushing harder toward committing to that exercise routine. You lack the energy to meal prep ahead of time, which ensures you are consuming a healthy and balanced diet. You resort to quick and ready meals and lounging on the couch. Countless hours of unproductive, wasted time is lost when you do not invest those crucial hours in sleeping. We both have been guilty of sacrificing sleep hours to gain productive work hours, and the trade-off is a heavier price to pay than we imagined.

The time to reign in your physical and mental health to supercharge your life is now, and we will show you how by invigorating your daily routines!

Routines rule our daily lives from the moment we wake up and stretch to the moment we hit the pillow yawning. So many of our behaviors and actions happen without thought because we are so accustomed to the routines we overlook. Sometimes this is great, like when your feet walk themselves home after a long shift so your mind can wander peacefully, but at other times routine can take over your life and prevent you from making necessary changes to your lifestyle or trying something new. They make us feel comfortable, but they can also trap us if they aren't occasionally refreshed or revamped to make room for new healthy routines. It's time to focus on building routines that will help you change your life and put you on the path to a healthier body and mind to being the best version of yourself.

ROUTINES

Routines are actions done at certain times or in a particular order, usually repeated daily or weekly. Your whole day is constructed around a series of routines within your routine. We have routines for everything, including morning routines, commuting to work or school, cleaning and cooking, shopping, showering, and going to bed. There are many benefits to keeping up with routines.

They can help us to stay organized and productive and assist us in completing tasks we would otherwise forget or procrastinate. They encourage you to achieve tasks and goals by setting aside time for them. Routines give structure to your day, so you can plan how to use your precious free time rather than wasting it, and having a system helps to create a calm environment because you know what to expect from your day.

When it comes to health, routines are instrumental in keeping up healthy habits and reaching your fitness goals:

- Routines help with stress management, reducing anxiety and heart disease risk.
- Morning and bedtime routines help to regulate your sleep cycle, improving your sleep hygiene and health and enabling you to wake up energized, with your body and mind rested and ready for the day.
- You can build healthy habits into your routine, like planning your trips to the grocery store rather than popping to the store when you're hungry, and planning time for healthy snacks into your routine will stop you from grazing or craving unhealthy snacks.
- Daily routines that make time for exercise will make a tremendous difference in your weight loss or fitness journey! Budgeting your time to allow for exercise means you are less likely to skip a

workout and won't feel like you have to rush through it.

- Incorporating meal planning into your routine will help you to eat a healthier diet because you can prepare for the day's meals in advance, rather than needing a quick-fix dinner—which often ends up being less than healthy—at the last moment.

Level Up Your Daily Routine

You can change up your daily routine at any time to make your day more productive or energizing—even small changes can make a huge difference as long as you commit. Here are some quick ideas to add to your daily routine to bring you a step closer to a healthy, happy, and balanced life.

Get Energized

Power up your day and get out of a slump with these routine rechargers:

- Drink a glass of room temperature water with a fresh lemon slice when you wake up—it will help improve digestion and refresh your body by removing toxins; while also giving you a boost of vitamin C.
- Work out in the morning to get your blood flowing and your muscles full of energy.

- Eat a nutritious breakfast every day.
- Stay hydrated by ensuring to drink plenty of water throughout your day.
- Eat an energizing lunch—avoid fatty foods, which can cause lethargy, and have a good dose of slow-release carbohydrates to get you through the afternoon.
- Stretch out the mid-afternoon slump! Our energy levels tend to drop around 3-4 p.m., so set up reminders to get up and stretch or take a quick walk when you feel the slump coming.
- Ditch the caffeine after 5 p.m.
- Have your dinner planned in advance so you can quickly throw together a healthy evening meal.
- Have another lemon water before going to bed at a reasonable hour.

Get Organized

Use these tips to bring a little more order and control to your busy life:

- Make your bed when you get up so you're less likely to crawl back into it and start your day in an organized mindset.
- Prepare your exercise outfits, work clothes, and work or gym bag the night before and lay them out ready for the morning.

- Wipe up behind yourself. After your shower, give the bathroom surfaces a quick wipe, and during and after cooking, do the same in the kitchen. Little and often cleaning is much easier than a big weekly clean that takes up half the weekend.
- Put things back where they belong when you're finished with them.
- Keep a grocery list on your fridge and add to it when you notice something is low so that you don't miss anything.
- Run an essential items check before you leave the house. Have you got your phone, keys, wallet, charger, employee ID, water bottle, etc.? Do this check every time you head out, and it will soon become a great habit.
- Prioritize your most important and urgent tasks for the day or week, and work your way through them first.
- Check your finances every morning and track your budget throughout the day.
- Do the dishes straight after dinner!

Be Productive

You can have a productive day every day if you shape your routine to work to your benefit!

- Plan your day the night before.
- Keep to the same bedtime and wake-up time every day.
- Declutter your workspace at the end of every day so that the next morning it is clear of distractions.
- Focus on your goals and priorities in the morning when your brain is most active and creative. Save emails and mind-numbing work for the afternoon.
- Tackle the most complex or the most urgent task first!
- Make time to *rest*—you could schedule a meditation or reading time in the afternoon to avoid burnout.
- Split your working day into 45-minute work sessions with 15-minute breaks between. Switch to another task for a while when you feel unproductive with a particular task.

Taking on all these habits may be overwhelming, so try slowly integrating them into your daily routine, one or a few at a time. One of the main reasons people struggle to keep to a routine is they make it too difficult or too packed with things to remember that they slip back into the easy old habits that weren't working for them either. Your routine shouldn't be so strict or cumbersome that when you miss a step, you feel like you have failed, as this can set up a negative mindset about your routine, making it more likely you won't keep to it. The key is to find balance in your routines to allow flexibility, set easy-to-follow patterns, and keep your routines realistically achievable.

Sticking to a Routine

Sticking to a new routine can be very challenging at first. You have to learn new behaviors and exercise your self-control more than you have been, which can make your new routine seem like more effort than it is worth. With time and perseverance, you'll find your routine easier and more rewarding, but how can you stick to it in those first few difficult weeks when it seems like your routine rules your every waking moment?

Firstly, it is fundamental to **remember *why* you changed your routine**. Keeping your initial motivations and goals in mind will keep you focused on the rewards for sticking to your routine and make the effort feel worthwhile. If you aim to create a productive weekday routine in order to be able to enjoy your weekends more, then keep that in mind when your to-do list seems daunting.

Next, **identify where you could improve the routine**. What area seems most arduous to maintain or integrate?

What part of your new routine keeps tripping you up? It may be that you find your unfamiliar early wake-up call a struggle or that you don't have time to cook the dinners you planned when you get home from work—find the weak spot and figure out a way to make it work rather than just giving up.

All the steps of your routine have a butterfly effect on each other, so if you start your day by waking up later than usual, it pushes back your whole day and can leave you rushing to finish tasks and playing catch-up. This in itself leads to added stress and demotivation, so the best way to stick to your routine is to **start the day on the front foot**. A good start makes a good day more likely!

Set a goal for sticking to your new routine. Set your plan that you'll keep laboring at it for two weeks. Check off the days you achieve it and track your progress to the end. If you miss a day, start over and see if you can do it for a solid two weeks the next time.

You can **keep a journal of how your new routine is working for you**. At the end of your busy day, wind down before bed by jotting down how your routine made you feel that day. What was strenuous, what really worked, and what are you hoping for the next day? Remind yourself of what your routine is working towards, and explore your feelings about your progress. You could also write down some **positive affirmations about your routine**, for example, "My routine makes me feel excited for the day!" or "Today was a very productive and successful day, and tomorrow will be too!"

There are many ways to make your routine work flawlessly every day. Ultimately, it all comes down to your willpower, self-control, and desire to stick to it and enjoy the benefits. Set the wheels in motion to force your routine to work for you and strive toward achieving your goals because they are crucial to taking control of your life.

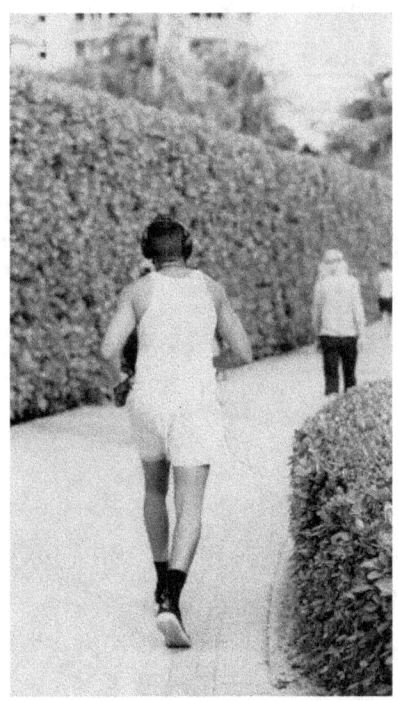

BUILDING THE BEST ROUTINE FOR THE BEST YOU

In a beautiful and uplifting article about struggling to stick to routines, Catherine Andrews wrote that "routines are an investment in yourself, and an act of self-love." (Andrews, 2018) When routines are viewed in this way, it is hard to find a reason *not* to invest in upgrading your routine to achieve your goals and improve your life. You deserve to enjoy the rewards and peace of mind of a healthy daily routine. After all, you work hard, and life is demanding enough without feeling unmotivated, distracted, and unproductive all the time. Seeing your routine as an act of self-love will help you to stick to it, knowing that you are gifting yourself time, energy, less stress, and better mental and physical health. You should be your own priority, and building a routine that prioritizes your health, goals, and values will improve your sense of self-worth and keep negative energy and influences out of your life.

Your routines should align your goals and direction across all areas, making time for fitness, reflection, self-care, and sleep. Think of each day of the week as a stepping stone to a better life. Every day should help you progress towards your goals, even if only in a tiny way, like sticking to your sleep schedule or taking the time to make a meal rather than ordering takeout. So, to build your new routines and daily schedule, keep your fitness, nutrition, and sleep goals in mind to ensure that you work towards them every day.

Let's build a goal-oriented routine for a 7-day stretch that could change your life in just a week! For each day, we'll add sleep, fitness, and nutrition elements—plus other areas—to gradually work up to a supercharged schedule one day at a time.

Sunday Night Checklist*

*For the week ahead, you'll need to get a notebook. Use half of the notebook to write your bedtime checklist, daily tasks, exercise plan, and meal plan, and the other half to keep a journal of reflections and notes on how the new routine works for you.

Start preparing for your new routine on a Sunday night, ready for the working week. Work through this checklist to get yourself in the perfect mindset for the changes and improvements to come!

1. After dinner, do the dishes straight away. Set a timer for 30 minutes and spend the time cleaning up the house, putting away laundry, and wiping down the kitchen and bathroom surfaces. Open your bedroom window and change your bed sheets.
2. Pour yourself a soothing cup of tea, take out paper and a pen, and make a list of the things

you need to do tomorrow. Then, put those things in order of importance so your tasks are prioritized—you'll be doing this exercise every night for the next week.

3. Next, plan your meals—breakfast, lunch, and dinner—for the whole next week, and make a grocery list. Include a few healthy snacks on the list. Go through your cabinets, fridge, and freezer to see what you already have in the house, and make use of that first!

4. Now plan an exercise session for 30 minutes each day, for example:

    a. Monday: Morning yoga (20 minutes), lunchtime walk (10 minutes)

    b. Tuesday: Morning Pilates (30 minutes)

    c. Wednesday: Morning jog (20 minutes), lunchtime yoga (10 minutes)

Give yourself two days when you take a gentle walk instead of a workout. You don't want to avoid exercise altogether, but "rest" days of low-intensity exercise will keep your body stronger than if you do nothing at all.

5. Prepare your exercise and work clothes for the morning and pack your work bag. Put a glass of water by your bed.

6. Around 9.30 p.m., start your sleep hygiene routine.

This Sunday night routine will kickstart the whole week to come and sets up some good habits from the beginning!

7-Day Supercharge

Use this routine as a template for every day this week—you can add and change things for each day, such as your exercises and meals, but it should keep to a similar order to help you build up good habits.

Morning:

- 7 a.m.: Wake up and have a quick stretch in bed. Don't lie around scrolling through social media—get straight up!
- Drink some water with fresh lemon.
- Do 20-30 minutes of exercise.
- Have a quick shower and dress for work.
- Eat a nutritious breakfast, e.g., oatmeal, scrambled eggs, or fruit and yogurt.
- Prepare a healthy lunch to take to work, ideally something with protein to aid concentration.
- Now you can check your phone and go to work!

Afternoon:

- At lunchtime, try to get in 10-15 minutes of gentle exercise—go for a walk, do some quick cardio exercises, or stretch at your desk.
- Eat your lunch and drink water.
- **Monday:** On your way home from work, do a food shop for everything you'll need for the week's meals.

Evening:

- Prepare and eat your dinner.
- Do the dishes and wipe down the kitchen.
- Spend an hour working towards one of your career, personal growth, or spiritual goals, or if you didn't have time for morning exercise, now is the time to do it!
- Now you can unwind with some TV or a hobby.
- Have a quick clean up and open the bedroom window.
- Write down your tasks for tomorrow, and set out your work clothes and bag.
- In your journal, write about how your new routine feels each day. Was it fun? How did it make you feel? How did your day improve? What changes felt easiest or most meddlesome? Take some time to reflect.

Bedtime:

- Start your sleep hygiene routine around 9.30 p.m.

  - Dim all the lights, and put on some soothing music.
  - Take a warm bath or shower.
  - Do your skincare routine and get into your pajamas.
  - Set your alarm for 7 a.m. and then turn off your phone wifi, lower your phone screen brightness, and put your phone on the other side of the room across from your bed.
  - Get into bed with a book and read for at least half an hour—if you choose a book that aligns with one of your goals, even better!
  - Drink some water.
  - Turn off your light by 11 p.m.

The purpose of this routine is to incorporate all the elements of this book into your week, enabling you to meet your goals, break bad habits, and improve your mental and physical health. It makes time for every facet of the two pillars and fills your day with healthy habits promoting self-care, progress, and wellness. After a week of this routine, you should feel energized and productive and like you've started on the right path for the life and future you hope for. Sticking to this routine in the long term and, in time, expanding and improving it will be an incredibly considerable learning experience.

Now you're ready to start your new routine, all that remains is to commit to taking back control of your life and focusing your energy on strengthening the two essential pillars of existence so that they can support you in all your endeavors, adventures, hopes, and dreams.

BEFORE YOU PUT YOUR SNEAKERS ON...

If this book has helped you understand the connection between your physical and mental health, and inspired you to prioritize both in your daily life, we hope you can do us a favor and leave a quick review on Amazon.

Share your thoughts on the 7-day supercharge and let them know how it made you feel. We would love to hear how this easy-to-follow routine impacted everything from your mood to your sleep.

WANT TO HELP OTHERS?

Thank you for your support. We are so looking forward to someone reading your words and deciding that this is the day they will take their health into their hands and put an end to bad habits standing in the way of success.

Scan the QR code for a quick review!

CONCLUSION

Working to improve your mental and physical health, to strengthen and build upon your two pillars, is a lifetime commitment that will bring purpose, clarity, and confidence into your life. The two pillars are the source of your energy and potential. Throughout life, you will draw on them every single day to achieve your goals, enjoy your endeavors, and face your challenges—this is why keeping them and yourself strong, stable, and supported is the most important thing you can do.

Your mental health is your compass, your internal guide that tells you what you want and need, who you are, and who you could be, and with care and attention, it can be an endless source of strength and energy. There is no limit to what you can achieve if you take care of your mind and encourage happiness and mental stability in your life. Your physical health and your body are your toolkits for life, your vessel through thick and thin, and this vessel, like any other, must be cared for, kept clean, healthy, and strong to make journeys and face the world's weather. With self-love and care, your body will carry you through life and open up a world of energy and adventure. It will walk you along the beach, climb mountains, carry your children, and so much more, bringing you to the places and experiences that will fill your life with joy and excitement. Pay attention to how your body feels and give it what it *needs*, not what it *wants*, and keep working towards a fitter, stronger, healthier body and a more fulfilling and enjoyable life.

There may be days in the future when, no matter how excellent your routines or habits are or how well you've slept or eaten, you feel unmotivated, demoralized, or unproductive and have wasted all your effort and sunk back into your old patterns and habits. It happens to everyone, and it doesn't mean you have failed or wasted your efforts—one crummy day mustn't deprive you of a hundred good days! Believe in yourself! You know who you are and no one else can take that away from you.

Come back to this book and remind yourself that you *can* do it. You *can* keep moving forward with simple changes and a positive mindset. Go back to your to-do list and pick one thing to get done, or drop something that's overwhelming you and do a meditation or some self-care to help you reset and regroup within yourself. Be honest about what is working and not working for you, and keep finding ways to change and improve that draw you closer to your goals. The trials and temptations of our modern world are a constant challenge to our mental and physical health, but to rise to that challenge and overcome it will strengthen your two pillars and give you a firm base for building a rewarding and happy life.

The book may be over, but your journey is just beginning. It is never too late to take the reins of your life and get on track to a better life and a better you. Taking back control of your life by breaking bad habits, supercharging your routine, and improving your mental and physical health takes courage, determination, and strength of will. By simply seeking a path to a better life, you have decided to put yourself first and gift yourself the life you deserve. You deserve to enjoy the rewards for your efforts, achieve your goals and dreams, and build an extraordinary life of adventure and joy. So, what are you waiting for? Get out there and use your new knowledge and skills to reinvigorate your life!

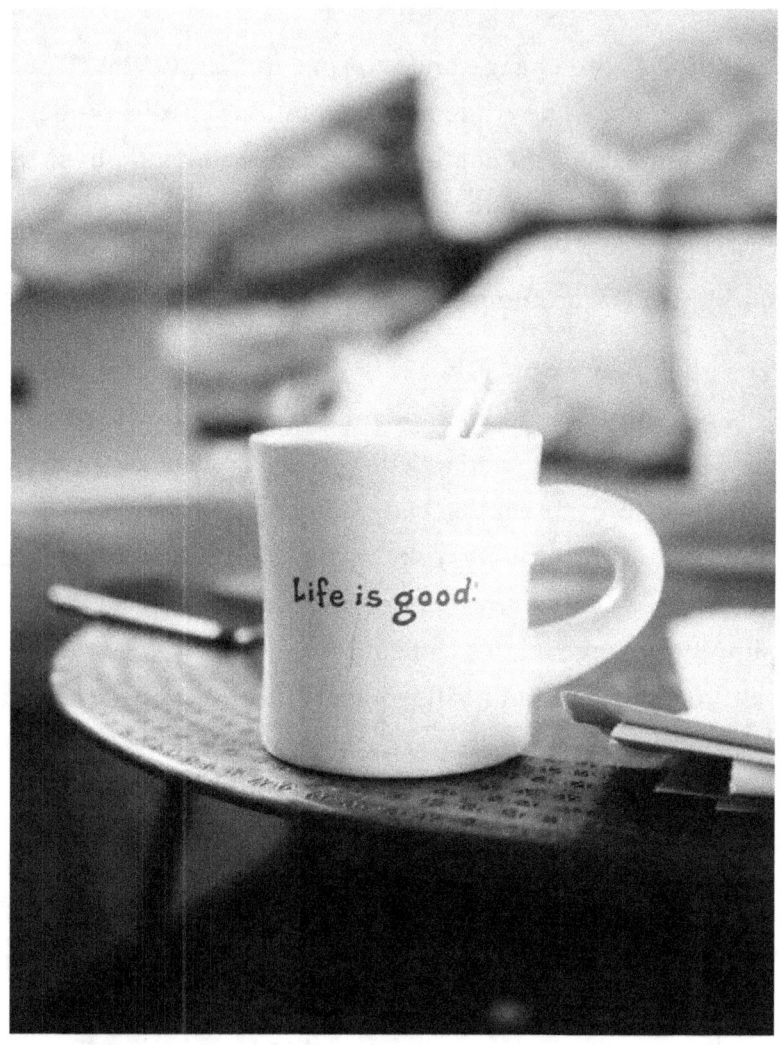

JUST FOR YOU!

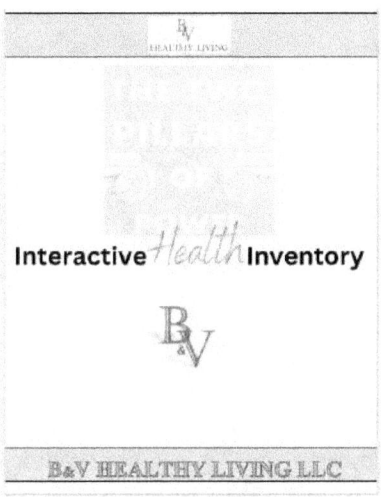

A FREE GIFT TO OUR READERS
Download and print the **Two Pillars of Power:**
Interactive Health Inventory

The Health Inventory should be used as you progress through each chapter assessing your current health and setting new goals that will transform your life right away! Visit the link:

https://bvhealthyliving.org/HealthInventory

REFERENCES

Altrogge, S. (2022, December). *12 morning and evening routines that will set up each day for success.* Zapier. https://zapier.com/blog/daily-routines/

Andrews, C. (2018, May 7). *I used to struggle with routines until I figured this out.* Medium. https://candrews.medium.com/struggling-with-sticking-to-routines-it-might-be-for-a-different-reason-than-you-think-e0378828182

Aronov-Jacoby, S. (2022, January 27). *The benefits of self-awareness.* Humber River Hospital. https://www.hrh.ca/2022/01/27/the-benefits-of-self-awareness/

Bennett, J. (2022, December 20). *This room-by-room guide makes deep cleaning your house so much easier.* Better Homes & Gardens. https://www.bhg.com/homekeeping/house-cleaning/tips/how-to-deep-clean-your-house/

Betz, M. (2022, September 14). *What is self-awareness, and why is it important?* BetterUp. https://www.betterup.com/blog/what-is-self-awareness

Bhatt Patel, R. (2021, July 16). *6 unexpected ways decluttering can help you destress, calm down, and take care of your mental health.* Apartment Therapy. https://www.apartmenttherapy.com/mental-health-benefits-decluttering-36948599

Bjarnadottir, A. (2021, November 2). *25 simple tips to make your diet healthier.* Healthline. https://www.healthline.com/nutrition/healthy-eating-tips#TOC_TITLE_HDR_10

Boksic, B. (2014, March 24). *What is a routine? 9 ways to define a routine that works.* Lifehack. https://www.lifehack.org/articles/productivity/why-using-routines-will-make-you-more-productive.html

Boulos, Dr. M. (2020, May 21). *Your healthy sleep checklist.* Heart and Stroke Foundation of Canada. https://www.heartandstroke.ca/articles/your-healthy-sleep-checklist

Brennan, D. (2021, March). *How does mental health affect physical health.*

WebMD. https://www.webmd.com/mental-health/how-does-mental-health-affect-physical-health

CDC. (2021, January 4). *How does sleep affect your heart health?* Centers for Disease Control and Prevention. https://www.cdc.gov/blood pressure/sleep.htm

CDC. (2022, September 13). *Sleep hygiene tips - sleep and sleep disorders.* Centers for Disease Control and Prevention; Centers for Disease Control and Prevention. https://www.cdc.gov/sleep/about_sleep/ sleep_hygiene.html

Centers for Disease Control and Prevention. (2022, June 16). *Benefits of physical activity.* Centers for Disease Control and Prevention; CDC. https://www.cdc.gov/physicalactivity/basics/pa-health/index. htm#:

Cherry, K. (2023, March 10). *What Is self-awareness?* Verywell Mind. https://www.verywellmind.com/what-is-self-awareness-2795023

Clear, J. (2013, May 13). *How to break a bad habit (and replace it with a good one).* James Clear. https://jamesclear.com/how-to-break-a-bad-habit

Covey, S. R. (2004). *The / habits of highly effective people: Powerful lessons in personal change.* Free Press.

Eatough, E. (2021, December 7). *How to form good habits (and ditch bad ones)* BetterUp. https://www.betterup.com/blog/building-habits

Eurich, T. (2018). *What self-awareness really is (and how to cultivate it).* Harvard Business Review; hbr.org. https://hbr.org/2018/01/what-self-awareness-really-is-and-how-to-cultivate-it

Felman, A. (2020, April 19). *Health: What does good health really mean?* Medical News Today. https://www.medicalnewstoday.com/arti cles/150999#types

Ferreira, M. (2018). *6 essential nutrients: What they are and why you need them.* Healthline. https://www.healthline.com/health/food-nutri tion/six-essential-nutrients

Gomstyn, A. (2019). *Food for your mood: How what you eat affects your mental health.* Aetna; Aetna. https://www.aetna.com/health-guide/ food-affects-mental-health.html

Gordon, S. (2021, February 23). *Mental health benefits of cleaning and decluttering.* Verywell Mind. https://www.verywellmind.com/how-mental-health-and-cleaning-are-connected-5097496

Headspace. (n.d.). *Sleep hygiene tips.* Headspace. Retrieved June 19, 2023, from https://www.headspace.com/sleep/sleep-hygiene

Ho, L. (2018, March 5). *Powerful daily routine examples for a healthy and high-achieving you.* Lifehack. https://www.lifehack.org/677367/powerful-daily-routine

Homemakers. (2020, October 1). */ Benefits of a clean and organized home.* Homemakers.com. https://www.homemakers.com/blog/ideas-and-advice/7-benefits-of-a-clean-and-organized-home.html

Jones, R. (2023). 57 Self-Awareness quotes to Know Yourself Better. *Happier Human.* https://www.happierhuman.com/self-awareness-quotes/

Konga Fitness. (n.d.). Best exercise and mental health quotes to get you through the week. https://kongafitness.com/best-exercise-and-mental-health-quotes-to-get-you-through-the-week/

Keenan, M. (2022, December 1). *200+ Motivational Quotes To Inspire and Win 2023.* Shopify. https://www.shopify.com/blog/motivational-quotes

Kristenson, S. (2022, May 5). */ benefits of setting & achieving SMART goals.* Develop Good Habits. https://www.developgoodhabits.com/benefits-smart-goals/

Lim, S. (2020, May 8). */ things you should do when you fail to achieve your goals.* Stunning Motivation. https://stunningmotivation.com/fail-achieve-goals/

Marks, J. L. (2023, April 26). *How to clean your house if depression is getting in your way.* Everyday Health. https://www.everydayhealth.com/depression/clean-house-when-youre-depressed.aspx

Mayo Clinic. (2018). *Infectious diseases - Symptoms and causes.* Mayo Clinic. https://www.mayoclinic.org/diseases-conditions/infectious-diseases/symptoms-causes/syc-20351173

Mental Health Foundation. (2022, February 18). *Physical health and mental health.* Mentalhealth.org. https://www.mentalhealth.org.uk/explore-mental-health/a-z-topics/physical-health-and-mental-health#:

Milkman, K. (2021, November 29). *How to build a habit in 5 steps, according to science*. CNN. https://edition.cnn.com/2021/11/29/health/5-steps-habit-builder-wellness/index.html

Mind Tools. (2022). *SMART Goals*. Mind Tools. https://www.mindtools.com/a4wo118/smart-goals

Mueller, S. (2023, January 1). *How to (finally) break that bad habit*. Wired. https://www.wired.com/story/how-to-break-bad-habits/

National Eating Disorders Association. (2018a, February 22). *Warning signs and symptoms*. National Eating Disorders Association. https://www.nationaleatingdisorders.org/warning-signs-and-symptoms

National Institute of Mental Health. (2023, March). *Mental illness*. National Institute of Mental Health. https://www.nimh.nih.gov/health/statistics/mental-illness

News In Health. (2017, May 31). *The benefits of slumber* (H. Wein, Ed.). NIH News in Health. https://newsinhealth.nih.gov/2013/04/benefits-slumber#:

NHS. (2022, February 24). *8 tips for healthy eating*. NHS. https://www.nhs.uk/live-well/eat-well/how-to-eat-a-balanced-diet/eight-tips-for-healthy-eating/

NHSinform. (2022, August 26). *Chronic pain*. NHSinform. https://www.nhsinform.scot/illnesses-and-conditions/brain-nerves-and-spinal-cord/chronic-pain#:

Page, S. (2021, February 8). 27 Inspirational Health Quotes to Motivate Employees. *Employee Wellness Blog*. Retrieved July 23, 2023, from https://info.totalwellnesshealth.com/blog/27-inspirational-health-quotes

Parker-Pope, T. (2020, February 18). *How to build healthy habits*. The New York Times. https://www.nytimes.com/2020/02/18/well/mind/how-to-build-healthy-habits.html

Perkal, Z. (2015, August 31). *30 ways to brighten your daily routine*. Wanderlust. https://wanderlust.com/journal/30-ways-to-brighten-your-daily-routine/

Pietrangelo, A. (2019, January 15). *How to be happy: 25 habits to add to your routine*. Healthline; Healthline Media. https://www.healthline.com/health/how-to-be-happy#daily-habits

Polar. (2019, June 18). *9 ways to make time for exercise with a busy sched-*

ule. Polar. https://www.polar.com/blog/9-ways-how-to-make-time-for-exercise/

Ra0, J. (2023, Jul6). *25 Awesome Quotes On Nutrition.* STYLECRAZE. https://www.stylecraze.com/articles/awesome-quotes-on-nutrition/

Raypole, C. (2019, October 29). *How to break a habit: 15 tips for success.* Healthline. https://www.healthline.com/health/how-to-break-a-habit#prepare-for-slipups

Riopel, L. (2019, September 14). *1/ self-awareness activities and exercises (+ test).* Positive Psychology. https://positivepsychology.com/self-awareness-exercises-activities-test/#questions

Saber Healthcare. (2021, March 9). */ ways to improve your diet & nutrition.* Saber Healthcare. https://www.saberhealth.com/news/blog/improve-your-nutrition

Scallon, T. (2020, June 26). *Essential nutrients.* St. Luke's Health. https://www.stlukeshealth.org/resources/essential-nutrients#:

Selhub, E. (2022, September 18). *Nutritional psychiatry: Your brain on food.* Harvard Health Blog; Harvard Health Publishing. https://www.health.harvard.edu/blog/nutritional-psychiatry-your-brain-on-food-201511168626

Semeco, A. (2017, February 10). *The top 10 benefits of regular exercise.* Healthline. https://www.healthline.com/nutrition/10-benefits-of-exercise#TOC_TITLE_HDR_11

Sherrell, Z. (2021, November 30). *5 neurological disorders: Symptoms explained.* Medical News Today. https://www.medicalnewstoday.com/articles/neurological-disorders

Sievers, M. (2020). 101 of the best sleep quotes + wall prints. *Casper Blog.* https://casper.com/blog/sleep-quotes/

Sleep Center of Middle Tennessee . (2019, April 4). *Get better sleep tonight with simple bedroom "spring cleaning."* Sleep Center of Middle Tennessee. https://sleepcenterinfo.com/blog/bedroom-spring-cleaning/#:

SokyaHealth. (2021, January 7). *Good nutrition for mental and physical health.* SokyaHealth. https://www.sokyahealth.com/thrive/the-importance-of-good-nutrition-for-mental-and-physical-health/

Stutter Health. (2019). *Eating well for mental health.* Sutterhealth.org.

https://www.sutterhealth.org/health/nutrition/eating-well-for-mental-health

Suni, E. (2020, August 14). *What is sleep hygiene?* (N. Vyas, Ed.). Sleep Foundation. https://www.sleepfoundation.org/sleep-hygiene

Suni, E. (2021, December 2). *Stages of sleep: What happens in a sleep cycle* (N. Vyas, Ed.). Sleep Foundation. https://www.sleepfoundation.org/stages-of-sleep

Suni, E., & Dimitriu, A. (2020, September 18). *Mental health and sleep.* Sleep Foundation; Sleep Foundation. https://www.sleepfoundation.org/mental-health

Thomas, A. (2022, April 19). *Dangers of diet culture.* Norman Regional Health System. https://www.normanregional.com/blog/dangers-of-diet-culture

Wild, M. (2018, June 8). *How to design your kitchen to eat Healthier - Debbie Rodrigues.* Debbie Rodrigues. https://debbieinshape.com/how-to-design-your-kitchen-to-eat-healthier/

Williams, T. (n.d.). *Bad habits: Definition, examples, and how to break them.* The Berkeley Well-Being Institute. Retrieved June 24, 2023, from https://www.berkeleywellbeing.com/bad-habits.html

World Health Organization. (2022, June 8). *Mental disorders.* World Health Organization. https://www.who.int/news-room/fact-sheets/detail/mental-disorders

Wix Answers *(2022, January 6). 50 inspiring quotes on business growth and Success. WIX Answers.* https://www.wixanswers.com/post/business-growth-quotes

Yuko, E. (2023, January 24). *12 home decor tips for a mental health boost.* Real Simple. https://www.realsimple.com/home-decor-for-mental-health-7098644#:

IMAGE REFERENCES

All images sourced on Unspla

The Two Pillars of Power

10 Life-Altering Steps to Confront Body
Image Anxiety and Eating Disorders

B&V Healthy Living

Trigger warning: This book contains references to eating disorders and mental illness. Please read with care and compassion.

Introduction

When you look in the mirror, do you struggle to find something you like about yourself? Do you obsess over your arms, your face, or other parts of your body? Do your "flaws" seem magnified in pictures or your mirror? Do you have a mean little voice in your head that judges your every action and puts you down for wearing something or eating something? Do you feel unable to accept yourself as you are, and are you constantly looking for ways to make your body "better?" These are all symptoms of body image issues and body dysmorphia, and no matter how long you have overlooked them, you're here now, which means you have recognized that you need help. You're tired of feeling awful about your body. All you want is to feel confident and happy in the body you have and not have your days ruled by anxiety and stress about how you look. You want to be able to eat and wear what you like without feeling terrible or like you've done something unforgivable—and you can. You've taken the first and most crucial step of all by simply picking up this book. You aren't going to suffer anymore, you aren't going to let your condition or body image issues rule your life—you want help, and you're going to get it. But how did things get so bad?

We live in a society obsessed with image. Every day, we are bombarded with more information on how to look better, dress better, eat better, and be a better version of ourselves if we only buy this or try that. Movies, media, and the internet fill almost every second of our time, splashed across our screens at work, on the way to work, at home, and even in the bath. On these screens, you see an ever-changing series of fashion trends, fad diets, weight-loss technology and treatments, idealized bodies, and unrealistic image standards. It's impossible to keep up, and you can't help but wonder, *would my life be better if I looked differently?*

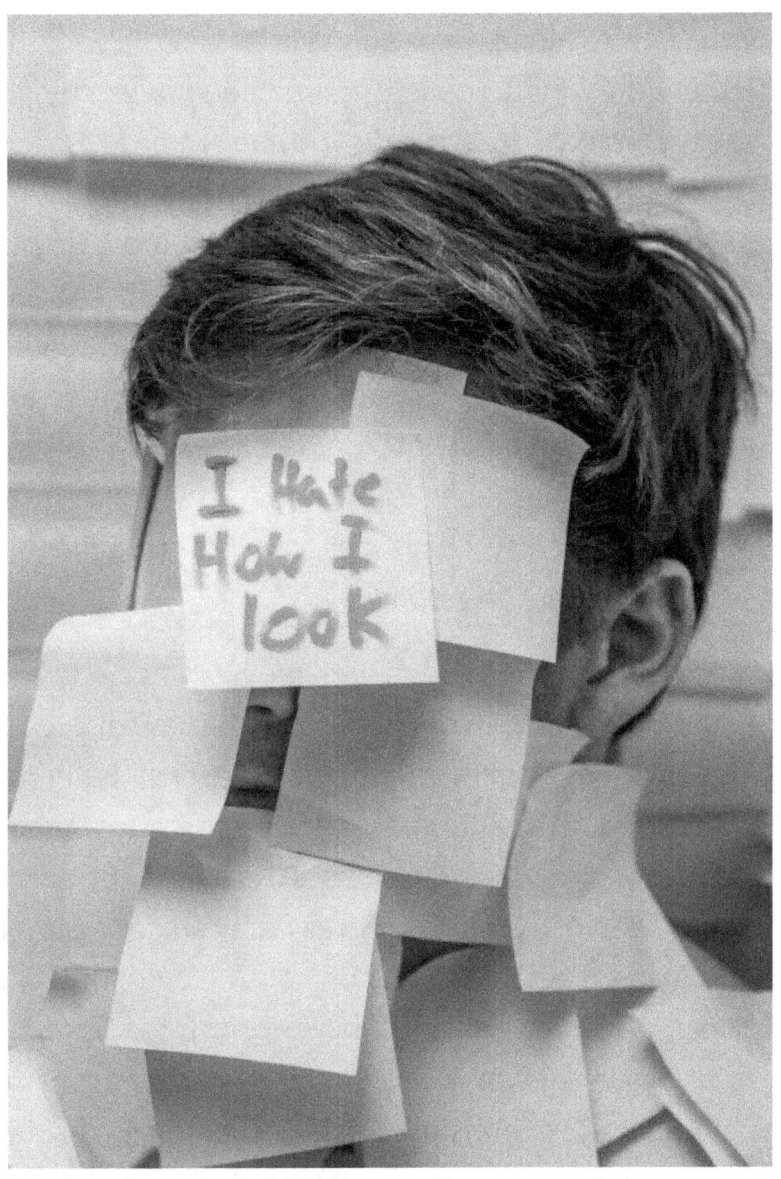

You're not alone in feeling as you do. Even the people on your screens, the people who seemingly set the standards, struggle with body image issues. Countless celebrities and artists throughout history have experienced body dysmorphia, some going to extreme lengths like cosmetic surgery to try and achieve the "perfect" image. From Sylvia Plath, Andy Warhol, and Britney Spears to, more recently, Lili Reinhart, Robert Pattinson, and Billie Eilish, everyone, no matter how great their life looks, how famous or pretty they are, can be struggling in secret to accept their body.

It isn't just the media and movies; body image issues like body dysmorphia and eating disorders can take root for a number of reasons. Bullying, trauma, racism, and peer pressure are all common causes of body dysmorphia, as are perfectionism and a fear of rejection. Stress and anxiety play a part, too. Feeling a lack of control over life and being in a constant state of worry can lead people to exercise control in any way they can by counting calories, overexercising, limiting food, and tracking their weight obsessively. Such behaviors are coping mechanisms, but while they feel helpful at the time, they are actually far more dangerous than they appear and can quickly lead to eating disorders.

Whether you have an eating disorder, you are conscious that you are developing one, or you know and love someone who is struggling with their body image, this book is here to take you through a journey to recovery.

This book will lay out your recovery journey in ten steps, with chapters on acknowledgment and acceptance, mindfulness and self-compassion, unraveling negative thought patterns, nourishment, coping mechanisms, self-love and self-care, growth and resilience, and ultimately, ways to embrace life, purpose, and future beyond recovery. Each chapter concludes with a targeted activity that will help you bring together and apply all that you have learned. These activities are designed to help you make positive progress and find a deeper understanding of your body image issues and mental health in a safe, supported, and self-guided way. You will learn how to navigate triggers and negative influences, develop healthy habits that promote self-love and healing, and find the confidence to reach out for support.

As part of the Two Pillars series, this book focuses on the impact of body image issues and body dysmorphia on the two major foundations of life: mental and physical health. Eating disorders and body dysmorphia have a significant effect on your body and mind, and overcoming them will bring balance back into your life. We are B&V Healthy Living, a husband and wife who have devoted their lives to helping people enjoy healthy and balanced lives based on the foundation of the Two Pillars of life. While we are not licensed medical profession-als, we have made it our mission to bring carefully curated information and guidance to people on how they can break free from bad habits and discover new ones that improve their quality of life by priori-tizing mental and physical health. We feel passion-ately that everyone deserves to live the life they dream of and that nothing should hold them back, especially not anxiety about their fantastic, incredi-ble, and unique bodies.

So, are you ready to take back your life from body image issues? Your recovery journey has begun.

Chapter 1
Step 1 - Acknowledging the Struggle

According to research, 28.8 million Americans will have an eating disorder during their lifetime (ANAD, 2021). There are a few types of eating disorders, and they often stem from body dysmorphia, which we will explore in this chapter. There is no specific cause for body dysmorphia. As with most mental health disorders, there are a range of factors in play, including genetics, social pressure, chemical imbalances, life experience, and trauma. Any person of any age, race, gender identity, sexuality, or social background can be affected by body dysmorphia. It infiltrates your life in many ways, from your daily decision-making about what to wear, eat, or do to your work, school, and social life. For many people with body dysmorphia, every day is spent feeling anxious, uncomfortable, and distracted by the nagging thoughts and emotions that come with it. While other people can relax and live in the moment, you feel on edge, waiting for someone to say or do something that confirms your negative perceptions about yourself. Let's delve deeper into body dysmorphia and begin your recovery journey.

Anxiety and Body Dysmorphia

What is Body Dysmorphia?

Body dysmorphic disorder (BDD) is a mental health condition in which you perceive or imagine flaws and defects in your appearance to such an extent that you can't stop thinking and worrying about them—sometimes for several hours a day—and eventually, your perceptions impact your ability to function and live a healthy life. The way you think about your body causes you terrible distress and anxiety, makes you embarrassed or ashamed of your body, and even leads you to try to fix your "flaws" with extreme methods like cosmetic procedures and obsessive dieting.

It's common for people suffering from body dysmor-phia to fixate on certain parts of their body, particu-larly the face, teeth and lips, stomach, hair, breasts, genitalia, and muscle size and tone. While everyone considers their appearance every day and makes diet and exercise choices based on it, body dysmorphia takes it a step further: Your perception of your body draws your focus to the point of obsession and drives every choice you make to excess, to such an extent that it has a significantly negative impact on your daily life, going so far as to interfere with your relationships, work, education, and, most of all, your health.

Signs of Body Dysmorphia

People struggling with body dysmorphia can be very good at concealing it, and we live in a world obsessed with appearance, so it may be hard to see when someone is more concerned about their appearance than usual, so look out for signs and symptoms such as

- preoccupation with a flaw or defect that others don't see or consider a problem—you might think you are out of proportion or the "wrong" shape, disfigured in some way, or that an area of your body is the wrong color or texture

- the belief that a physical flaw or defect makes you ugly
- the belief that people are mocking you or talking about you negatively because of your appearance
- obsessive or compulsive behavior and rituals aimed at fixing or hiding perceived flaws, such as

  - skin picking
  - constantly checking the mirror
  - over-exercising and targeting exercise at certain body features
  - frequently weighing yourself
  - heavily editing photos of yourself
  - buying fad products and treatments regularly

- using clothes and makeup specifically to hide perceived flaws
- constantly seeking reassurance about your appearance or comparing your appearance to others
- avoiding situations where perceived flaws may be on display, like swimming, sports, dining out, or clothes shopping

Anxiety's Role

Anxiety is both a symptom and a consequence of body dysmorphia. The idea that your appearance dictates your worth or people's opinions about you can lead to crippling social anxiety and low self-esteem, and anxiety about your appearance is what sets off body dysmorphia. Everyone feels anxious about things—work, school, decisions, money—but when it comes to body image, anxiety can have detrimental consequences, leading you down a rabbit hole of negativity about yourself. Anxiety can cloud your ability to see reality, flooding you with fear and doubt and causing you to overthink. This is when you lose a sense of control, and obsessive thoughts and behaviors can easily set in as you attempt to find stability and regain your power. People with anxiety may fixate on their appearance as a defense mechanism or as a way of anticipating other people's comments and opinions. Anxiety is also linked with perfectionism, so someone with anxiety and body dysmorphia may set unrealistic and unattainable standards for their body.

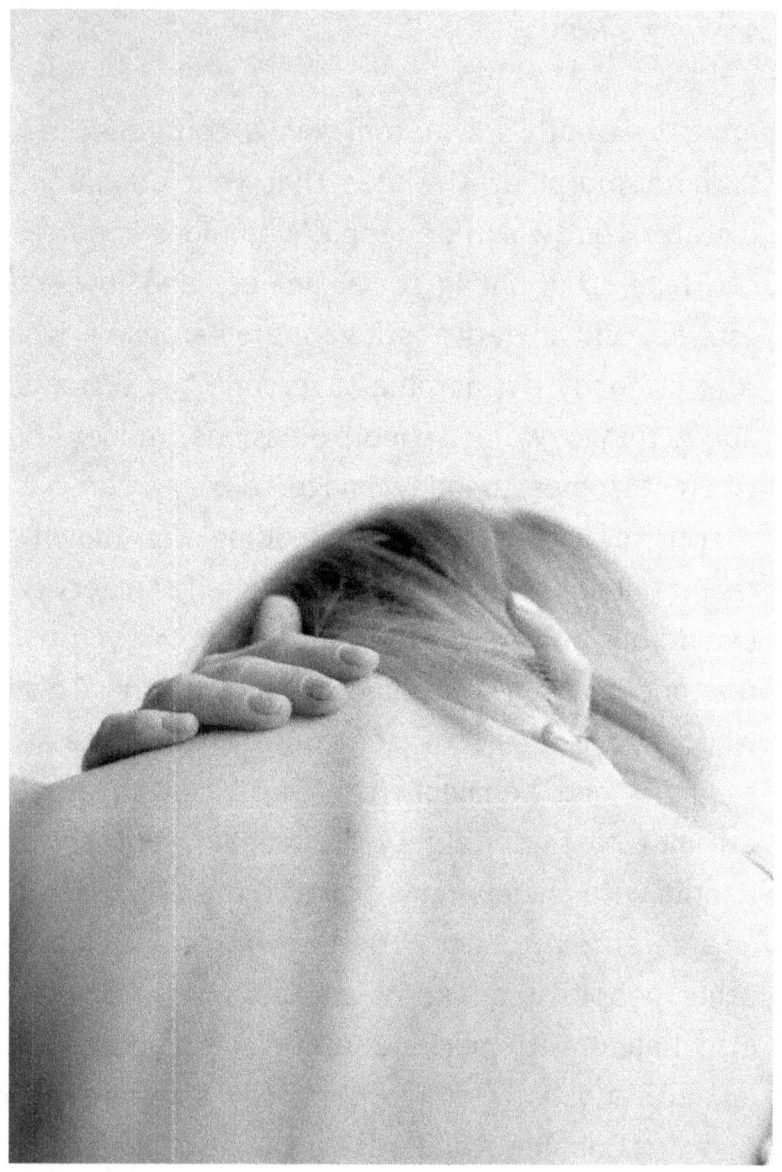

The Impact of Body Dysmorphia

Self-esteem, body image, and self-confidence are heavily impacted by body dysmorphia. People with BDD may be convinced they are unattractive, deformed, or unworthy because of their perceptions of their appearance, and this leads them to have a very negative view of themself, lowering their self-esteem. With low self-esteem comes a need for external validation, for others' reassurance about and validation of your appearance, and with this, the notion that your worth is actually tied to your physical appearance, as that is what people will comment on. This adds to your struggles as it encourages you to hyperfocus on maintaining the appearance that has been complimented, sometimes at the expense of your health and other priorities.

Seeking approval also comes with a fear of disapproval, which can lead someone with body dysmorphia to avoid social situations that might draw attention to their perceived flaws—such as swimming pools, playing sports, or going clothes shopping—for fear of getting negative comments and having their fears validated. People with BDD can struggle terribly with isolation, cutting themselves off from friends and family as a defense mechanism, leaving them alone with their negative thoughts about themselves, which further harms their self-esteem. Being alone also means you don't see the positive impact you have on other people and how much they enjoy your company and value your friendship, which could give you a huge boost in self-esteem.

Perfectionism is closely linked to anxiety, and for people with BDD, it can make things very difficult. It encourages them to set high and often unrealistic and unattainable standards for their body, which in turn increases the pressure they put on themselves and their dissatisfaction with their body when it can't meet their standards. This perfectionism can lead to obsessive behavior in an attempt to control the body and sometimes to cosmetic procedures to permanently banish perceived flaws.

Confidence is always a casualty of body dysmorphia. You may not feel you can dress or socialize with confidence because of your anxiety about your body, and you may also try to deflect attention from yourself by hiding in a crowd, not speaking, or simply avoiding people and places altogether. This affects the way people perceive you and doesn't show your true self, which can harm your self-image and exacerbate feelings of isolation, anxiety, and unworthiness.

When you feel your self-worth is intrinsically tied to your physical appearance, it has a significant impact on your ability to function in daily life. You are more likely to pour your time, energy, and concentration into obsessing over your body rather than into your work and relationships, which can lead to underperforming and needing more support to meet the needs of your responsibilities. The sense of failure and anxiety that comes with this damages your mental health and holds you back from fulfilling your potential and achieving your goals.

Body dysmorphia can have a severe and harmful impact on your mental and physical health, causing problems such as

- depression
- misuse of alcohol and drugs
- eating disorders
- obsessive-compulsive disorder (OCD)
- self-harm and suicidal thoughts

Acknowledgment and Acceptance

The first and possibly most crucial step in your journey to overcome body dysmorphia is to acknowledge your struggle, understand the challenges you are facing, and, with understanding, make your problem more approachable and actionable. Acceptance develops over time, and the path to acceptance involves taking dynamic and purposeful steps to take an active role in your own life again rather than allowing your life to be ruled by your mental health.

Steps to Acceptance

1. **Acknowledge and validate your emotions:** Take the time to acknowledge your struggle and the emotions that come with that acknowledgment. It's common for people to feel ashamed or angry at themselves at the start of their journey, resenting their body and mind for being "weak," and it's okay to feel that way. Write down all the things you are feeling to help release them. Don't edit your emotions or try to justify them; just experience them and channel them to the page. Acknowledging how you feel will help you move forward from a place of honesty.

2. Educate yourself about your condition: Information is power, so research and explore your health condition to better understand what is happening to you, why it is happening, and the effect it has on your life. Look into what may have caused or triggered your condition, and piece together how you have arrived here.

3. Seek support and professional help: The battle may be waging inside you, but you don't have to fight it alone. Reach out to friends and family who you trust, who will be understanding, and who are in a position to support you in your struggles with your condition. These are your "safe" people. Approach a professional for medical advice and therapy to help you get on track to recovery in the healthiest way possible. You can also find a local support group in your area so you can help and be helped by others going through the same thing as you.

4. Practice self-compassion and avoid blame: You aren't to blame for what is happening to you, and you've been tough enough on yourself already, so now it's time to be gentle and kind to yourself. You are not your illness; it doesn't define who you are, so now is the time to reestablish your place in the world, find the fun and enjoyment in life again, and build a positive sense of self by affirming your strengths and taking back your identity.

5. **Be patient:** You can't rush recovery, and there will be setbacks and challenges in the future, but trust that you are always moving forward, learning, and growing stronger, and be patient with yourself, your body, and your journey. It will be worth it!

6. **Find healthy coping strategies:** Start building coping strategies—however small—into your daily life to help you get through everyday struggles. We'll revisit this area in-depth later on.

- Journal every day to free your thoughts and emotions.

- Call your "safe" people.

- Make a plan to meet your needs—if you live with someone else, make a plan together so they know how they can support and help you through their own actions.

- Practice positive self-talk. If you find yourself thinking negative thoughts about your body, speak a positive thought aloud to yourself instead.

- Start every day with a positive affirmation!

- Change the subject when people talk about body issues around you or ask them not to.

- Pamper your body.

- Plan enjoyable activities to refocus your attention on things you are passionate about.

- Pick up a new hobby to fill your time so you don't spend it overthinking.

- Change your routine to avoid triggers.

- Surround yourself with people who make you feel good!

7. **Set realistic expectations and celebrate your progress:** This is going to be a long and unpredictable journey, and everyone's recovery happens on a different timeline and in a unique way. You'll find your way, but keep your expectations realistic throughout the journey, and don't demand too much from yourself. Reward yourself for your progress, and celebrate your wins, however small they seem.

8. **Prioritize your well-being:** Now is the time to focus your efforts, energy, and time on yourself and banish anything from your life that negatively impacts you and interferes with your recovery— including friendships and bad habits.

Step 1 Activity: A Letter of Compassion

Your first activity requires only pen and paper. Write yourself a compassionate and understanding letter that acknowledges and validates your struggles with body dysmorphia. Be as gentle with yourself as you would with a loved one or even a child, and be honest and open with yourself about your thoughts and feelings. Let yourself know that you are supported and that it is time to move forward and seek help.

You could write about

- how you think you got to this point
- how you hope to move forward
- things you are looking forward to post-recovery
- what you can do to be healthier and happier
- how you are feeling about your body dysmorphia: Does it frighten or anger you? Write how you feel.
- seeing yourself: Tell yourself that you see your pain and that you love yourself. Validate yourself and your feelings.

When you are finished, read your letter aloud to yourself. You can read your letter back whenever you feel down or overwhelmed by your body dysmorphia.

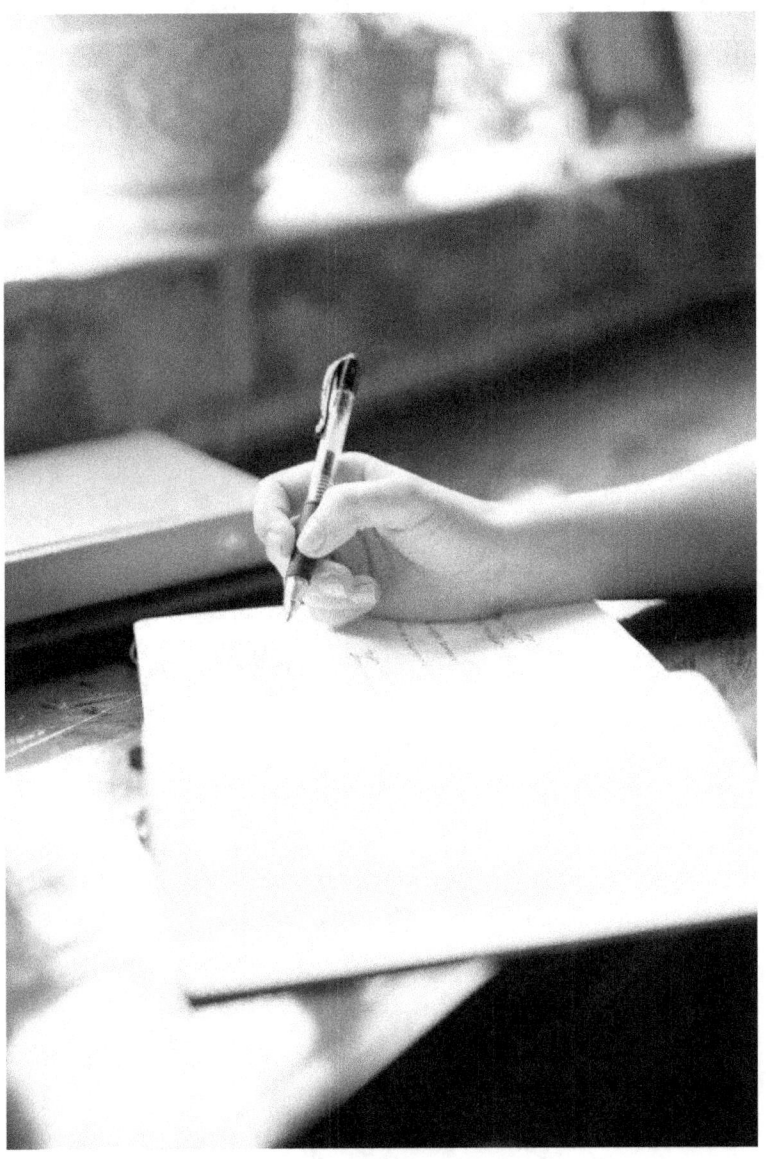

Seeking help is crucial—no one should have to fight their battles alone—and in the next chapter, you will explore how to approach getting help and deepen your understanding of body dysmorphia and the illnesses and disorders associated with it.

Chapter 2
Step 2 - Breaking the Silence and Seeking Help

Body dysmorphia can lead to eating disorders in an attempt to take control of your body and alter your appearance to align with your perception of an "ideal body." These eating disorders can quickly become damaging and have severe consequences on your health, and without help, you have little chance of overcoming them. There is a temptation to fight your battles alone that comes from anxiety and fear of other people's judgment and of being a burden on your loved ones, but hiding your condition can be isolating and make you feel more alone in your struggles. Seeking out and accepting help is an essential part of your recovery from body dysmorphia and eating disorders. While opening up is easier said than done, this chapter will help you understand why it is crucial to find the courage to do so.

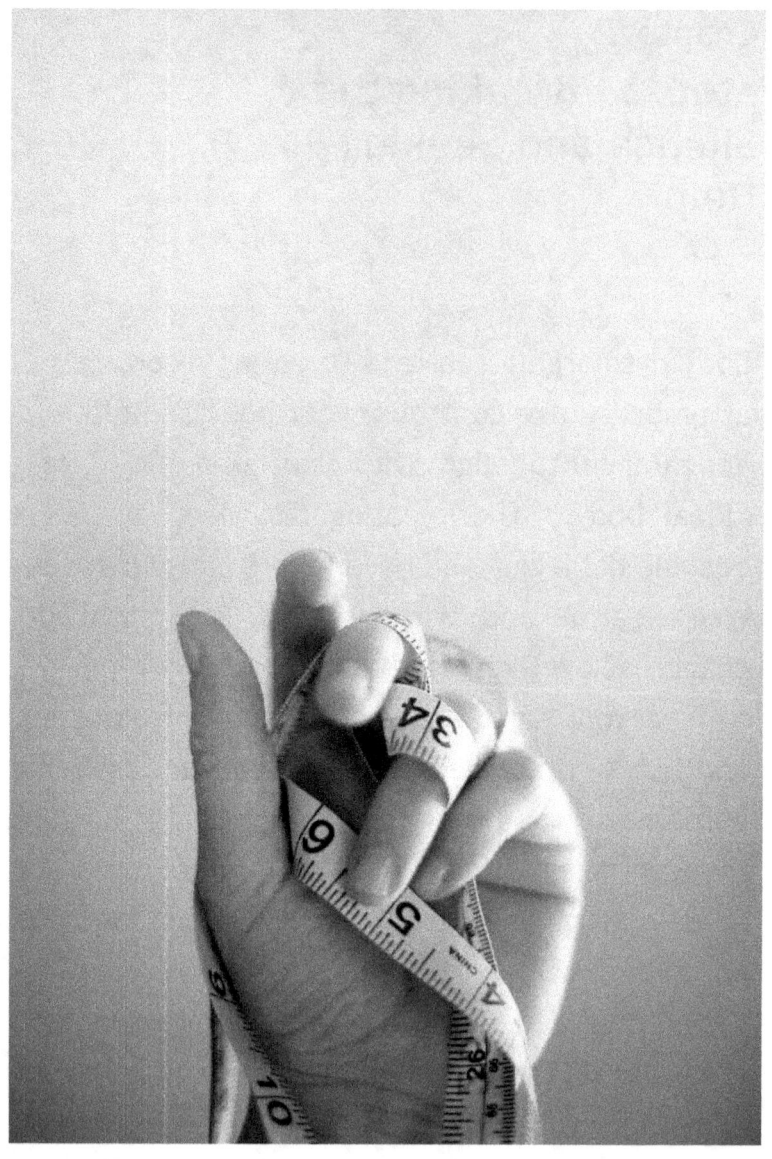

Eating Disorders

Eating disorders are complex and dangerous mental health conditions that cause unhealthy and obsessive eating habits that will have severe consequences if left untreated. They often start as an obsession with weight, food, or body image, leading to compulsive behaviors and symptoms like restriction of food, binges and purges of food, and overexercising. Eating disorders have an effect on people from all walks of life, often taking root during their teenage years. There are many kinds of eating disorders—and getting diagnosed correctly is vital to your recovery—but we'll look more closely at the signs, symptoms, and effects of some of the most common ones.

Anorexia

Perhaps the most well-known eating disorder of them all is Anorexia nervosa. Generally beginning during the teenage or early adulthood years, people with anorexia believe they are overweight no matter their size and will constantly monitor and try to reduce their weight, even if they are dangerously underweight already. They will likely eat a severely restricted diet, avoid certain foods entirely, fast for long periods of time, and exercise excessively. They may also purge what little they eat by throwing up or taking laxatives. Anorexia can severely damage the body, causing infertility, organ failure, and death if left untreated.

There are two subtypes of anorexia—restricting and binge eating/purging. People with restrictive anorexia lose weight by fasting, dieting, and exercising excessively. At the same time, those with the binge/purge type will either binge on large amounts of food at once or eat very little and, after that, will purge whatever they have eaten.

Symptoms of anorexia include:

- restricted eating habits
- fear of weight gain
- persistent behavior aimed at avoiding weight gain
- obsession with being thin or maintaining an unhealthy level of thinness
- heavy influence of body weight or shape on self-esteem and self-worth
- distorted perception of body image
- insistent denial of being underweight
- obsessive-compulsive behavior regarding food, e.g., collecting low-fat/low-carb

recipes, weighing, counting, and hoarding
food
- avoiding mealtimes and eating in public or
around other people, even family
- demonstrating a need to control their
environment and everything they consume

Bulimia

Bulimia nervosa is another common and well known
eating disorder, again frequently starting during
teenage years. People with bulimia tend to eat enormous amounts of food, often in a specific amount of
time. They will eat until they are painfully full,
feeling that there is no way to stop or control how
much they eat. These food binges often consist of a
food they would usually avoid or highly restrict. After
binging, they will attempt to purge the food in order
to compensate for the calories they have eaten and
to relieve gut discomfort by vomiting, fasting, taking
laxatives or diuretics, or exercising excessively.

From the outside, bulimia can be harder to spot than
anorexia since people with bulimia may maintain a
typical weight rather than lose a great deal and will
often hide their bulimic behavior by binging and
purging in secret. The effects of bulimia are as

damaging as those of anorexia, sometimes causing severe dehydration, kidney problems, strokes, and heart attacks. Often, those with bulimia will experience an inflamed, swollen, or sore throat, swollen glands, tooth decay, acid reflux, gut irritation, and hormonal imbalances.

Symptoms of bulimia include:

- recurring episodes of binge eating without control
- purging behavior to prevent weight gain
- body image-influenced self-esteem and self-worth
- fear of weight gain
- secretive or avoidant behavior around food
- frequent trips to the bathroom after eating

Binge Eating Disorder

The most common eating disorder, and an increasingly common illness among teenagers and young adults, is Binge eating disorder. People who suffer from binge eating disorder eat large and uncontrolled amounts of food in a short amount of time and will feel they cannot stop until they are full to the point of pain. They don't restrict or purge to compensate for their binge eating and will often make unhealthy nutrition choices, choosing to binge foods high in sugar, fats, and calories. This makes them particularly vulnerable to obesity-related medical conditions like heart disease, diabetes, and strokes.

Symptoms of binge eating disorder include:

- devouring large quantities of foods quickly without control, despite feeling full or not hungry, and sometimes in secret

- hoarding and hiding stores of food
- feeling ashamed, disgusted, or guilty when thinking about binge eating behavior

- not purging after a binge

Avoidant/Restrictive Food Intake Disorder

Avoidant/restrictive food intake disorder (ARFID) can begin in childhood and appear at any time throughout life. It usually manifests as disturbed eating patterns caused by a distaste for or inability to eat foods of particular tastes, smells, colors, textures, and temperatures. It is more than "picky eating." As the list of foods refused grows, the more the person with ARFID's health is negatively affected until they cannot get the nutrients their body needs to grow and stay healthy.

Symptoms of ARFID include:

- nutrient deficiencies resulting in a dependence on supplements or even tube feeding
- avoidant or restrictive eating that severely limits calories and nutrient intake
- weight loss and frequent illness
- poor development for age and height

Other Eating Disorders

There are other eating disorders, including pica, rumination disorder, night eating syndrome, and many more that are categorized as other specified feeding or eating disorders (OSFED).

One that falls in this category and is a growing concern is orthorexia. People with orthorexia are obsessive about healthy eating and may compulsively check ingredients and nutritional labels on foods and obsessively follow social media accounts that promote a "healthy lifestyle." They can be prone to following fad diets, swapping between diets regularly, and eliminating food groups entirely for fear that they are unhealthy or because they believe or have been told that they are. They may experience severe weight loss and malnutrition, struggle to eat around others, constantly worry over diets, and try to control their food intake excessively. For people with orthorexia, their diet influences their self-esteem and self-worth, and they measure their personal success and worth based on how well they comply with their diet and lifestyle rules.

Seeking Help

You must seek help if you think you or someone you know has an eating disorder. Without treatment, eating disorders can be damaging and even deadly and have long-term physical and mental health consequences. In order to treat an eating disorder, you need to determine the mental health issues that may have caused it, along with treating the physical health problems the eating disorder has caused. As a result, treatment for eating disorders is usually a combination of psychotherapy, medication, and nutritional counseling and education.

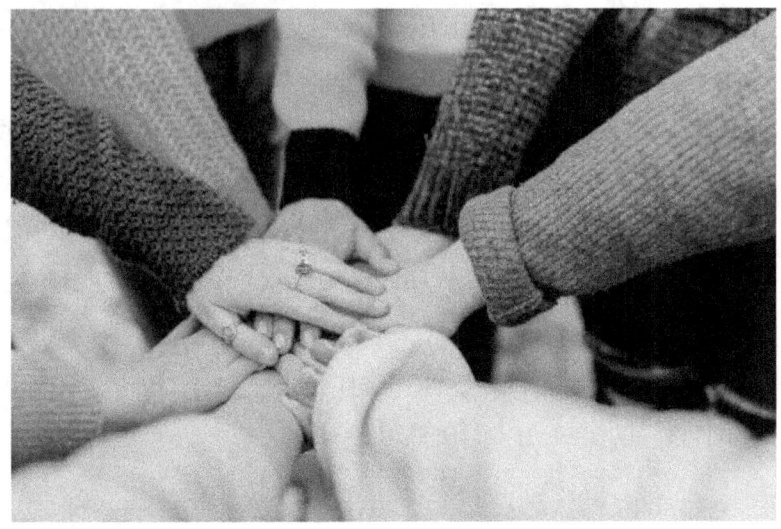

Your Treatment Team

Taking an organized approach to your recovery can help you feel in control and help you manage your symptoms better. Start by confiding in someone you trust to open the conversation and take a little pressure off yourself. This will start the ball rolling, and now you have someone else in your corner to encourage and support you. Next, make an appointment with your doctor and speak to them about your condition and fears—they will refer you to specialists who will play an essential role in your recovery. Your treatment team will likely include the following:

- **Medical and dental specialists** to treat the physical problems caused by your disorder
- **Mental health professionals,** including a psychologist to provide therapy, and sometimes a psychiatrist if you need medication
- **A dietician** to help you build a diet plan and educate you about nutrition

People living with someone with an eating disorder should also take an active role in the recovery process by supervising mealtimes, tracking medication, and providing emotional support and encouragement.

Treatment can take a long time, and you may need to see your treatment team regularly, even once you start to make noticeable and positive progress. Your treatment team will work with you to make a treatment plan for your recovery that meets your needs and sets achievable goals and clear guidelines.

Your treatment plan will cover:

- treatment goals to keep you moving forward
- a plan to treat the physical and mental health issues caused by your disorder

- resources that are available in your area to help you keep to your plan and meet your goals.
- affordable treatment options: Hospitalization and outpatient programs can be expensive, even with insurance. Your treatment team will help you find ways to manage the financial responsibilities of your treatment and ensure that you get help no matter your financial situation

The road to recovery can be daunting, but the odds are in your favor with your team and loved ones behind you. Seeking help is a sign of strength, not weakness—facing the challenge and reaching out is the bravest and most vital thing you can do.

Stigma and Support

Reaching out for help is made more challenging by the stigma that surrounds eating disorders. A stigma is when people negatively see you because of your disorder or illness, using the disorder to label you and make judgments about you that have nothing to do with who you really are. Stigma has many harmful effects, including causing feelings of shame, self-doubt, and isolation, making people reluctant to seek help. Stigma can lead family and friends to be unsupportive and to bullying and harassment at work or school. Stigma can also lead you to miss opportunities at work or school for fear of drawing attention to yourself or for fear of failure and rejection. By hiding your disorder from the world, you hope to avoid the effects of stigma, but by doing this, you make it impossible to recover and get help.

People with eating disorders often struggle in silence because they are worried about what other people will say or think or how they will be treated differently if people know they have an eating disorder. A common fear is that they will be accused of "attention-seeking", "fishing for compliments", or forced or shamed into eating. These kinds of negative attention and lack of understanding make it very difficult to have an open and honest conversation about your disorder.

You don't have to let stigma rule your recovery, though. Here are some ways to fight stigma and take control of your recovery narrative:

- **Educate yourself** about mental health conditions and eating disorders and the misconceptions associated with them. Knowledge will help you dispel the myths people have heard and aid you in promoting understanding. Be sure to use reputable and trusted resources for your information, like those listed below.
- **Challenge the secrecy** of stigma by speaking openly and honestly about your struggles and disorder, and if you feel comfortable, share your story with others to help them open up, too. Mental illness is not a shameful secret!
- **Seek supportive environments** and connect with people who are supportive, understanding, and empathetic about the challenges of mental health and eating disorders. Environments where people can have open dialogue about their disorders, like support groups, are fantastic.
- **Use person-first language** when you are talking about mental health and eating disorders to emphasize that the person is not defined or labeled by their disorder. For example, don't say, "I'm bulimic," say, "I have bulimia" instead.

- **Seek professional help,** and don't allow fear of judgment to hold you back from doing so.
- **Remember, it's not personal.** People's judgments about you come from false information and a lack of understanding, not from personal knowledge of you. Once they get to know you, they'll believe very differently!
- **Speak up for yourself and others.** If you hear someone saying negative or incorrect things or see someone discriminating against someone, step in and stop them short. By showing your support for others and your ability to stand up for yourself, you are fighting against stigma.

Help Resources

Getting accurate and informed advice is essential to your recovery, so use the following resources to find the help, information, and support you need.

Mental Health

Substance Abuse and Mental Health Services Administration (SAMHSA) offers a free, confidential, 24/7, 365-days-a-year service for people or families dealing with mental health disorders.

Mental Health America (MHA) offers information, resources, toolkits, and a screening test to help you understand and identify your condition.

Mental Health First Aid

National Institute of Mental Health (NIMH)

Anxiety and Depression Association of America (ADAA) offers webinars and help finding a therapist, along with many other resources.

Body Dysmorphia and Eating Disorders

National Eating Disorders Association (NEDA)

National Association of Anorexia Nervosa and Associated Disorders (ANAD) is one of the top nonprofit organizations in the US for eating disorders, providing support groups, treatment resources, holding events, and a free helpline.

Families Empowered and Supporting Treatment of Eating Disorders (FEAST)

Body Dysmorphic Disorder Foundation offers an online test to help determine if you have BDD, plus expert advice, recovery stories, and lots of information.

Eating Recovery Center provides information and resources for all eating disorders.

Step 2 Activity: Open Up

Your task for this chapter is to open up. Identify at least one person you trust and feel comfortable talking to about your struggles. Share your experience and struggles with them, and ask for their support. They may have no idea that you are struggling, or they may surprise you by being relieved that you can talk to them after all. Offer them understanding in return, as they may struggle to hear and process what you say, and share some of the resources above with them to help you both take the next step toward recovery. You are not asking them to cure you, only for them to listen and care.

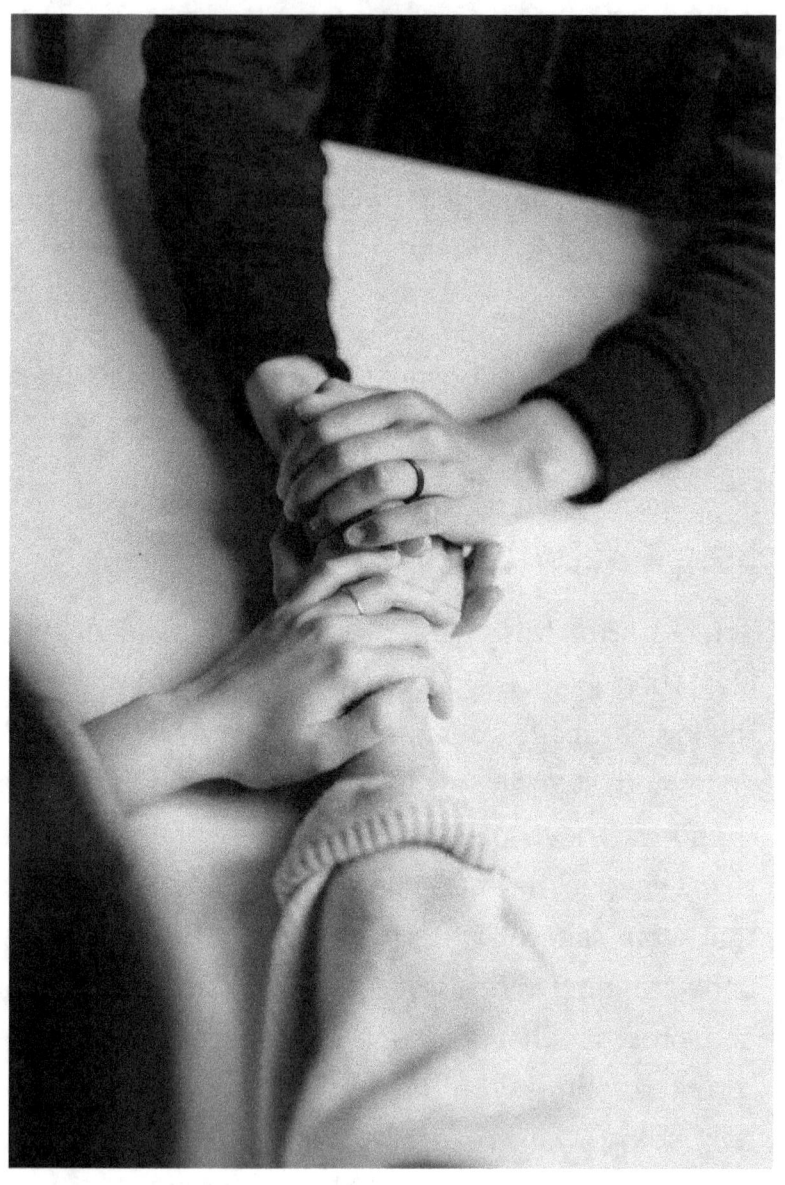

Compassion from others will be essential to your recovery, but self-compassion is even more critical. In the next chapter, you'll learn how to be kind to yourself again and break the negative thought cycles that are holding you back.

Chapter 3
Step 3 - Cultivating Self-Compassion and Mindfulness

After viewing your body in such a negative way, you'll have to relearn some self-compassion and self-acceptance in order to move forward through recovery. Healing the body begins with healing the mind and finding healthier and safer ways to view yourself and the world around you. Mindfulness is one of the greatest tools for recovery from mental health conditions. Practicing often will help you dig deeper into your mind and better understand your struggles, issues, and ideas about yourself. Self-compassion takes this understanding and enables you to use it to see yourself with a more positive and generous eye, encouraging you to demonstrate kindness to yourself as you would to others. With self-compassion and mindfulness, you can start to reclaim your mind from your condition and learn to love yourself again.

Developing Self-Compassion

Anyone struggling with an eating disorder or BDD has a tendency to judge themself harshly and be very self-critical, finding faults and flaws wherever they can and blaming themselves for mistakes even when it's not their fault. Harmful self-talk and a negative self-image have a detrimental effect on your self-worth and confidence, increasing stress, anxiety, and depression. However, if you can turn your mindset around and show yourself a little love and understanding, you'll see a massive difference in your approach to life, the future, your health, your body, and your mental health.

Self-compassion is choosing to recognize that you are doing your best given your circumstances and with the energy and knowledge you have and extending yourself patience, kindness, and grace, as you would to anyone else in your position. When we receive compassion from others, we feel safe, supported, calm, unjudged, and understood. Being able to give yourself those feelings is an essential part of living a healthy life and enjoying robust mental health.

Here are some ways to develop your self-compassion and build a strong foundation for your recovery.

- **Acknowledge your struggles and validate your feelings**. Remind yourself that it is okay to experience difficult thoughts and emotions, and do not judge yourself for your feelings.
- **Treat yourself with kindness**, as you would a friend or loved one if they were in your position.
- **Practice mindfulness and stay present.** Grounding yourself in the moment will keep you from being overwhelmed by past regrets and future worries and help you approach your mental health without judgment.
- **Seek support.** Reach out to friends, family, and professionals for support, and don't put off asking for help.
- **Set boundaries** that prioritize your needs, well-being, and self-care. Say "no" to anything that makes you uncomfortable or triggers you.

- **Focus on your needs.** Your body and mind need rest, nutrition, and exercise in order to function at their best, so make time for all of them.
- **Practice positive self-talk** to challenge negative thoughts and replace them with positive affirmations that boost your mood, confidence, and energy.
- **Forgive yourself** for your past actions and choices and accept that you must learn from them in order to grow.
- **Embrace your imperfections.** Nobody is perfect, and your flaws are what make you unique, interesting, and special.
- **Use self-compassion exercises** like writing a letter to yourself or recording voice affirmations to listen to when you are struggling.
- **Avoid comparisons.** Try not to compare yourself to other people, especially in terms of body image or mental health. Everyone is on their own journey, and you deserve support regardless of other people's experiences.

Managing Anxiety and Negativity with Mindfulness

Anxiety happens when your body is feeling too much stress and goes into fight-or-flight mode, putting you on alert and causing you to overthink and be overstimulated by fear. Body dysmorphia and eating disorders make anxiety worse because you are constantly in a state of stress, worrying about your body and what people think of it. Mindfulness is a fantastic way to manage your anxiety and any negative thoughts you have about your body. It forces you to be fully present and aware rather than in a reactive or passive state, focusing your attention inward and nonjudgmentally rather than on what is happening around you. Best of all, mindfulness allows you to explore your condition's complex emotions and underlying causes safely and openly rather than trying to fight against them.

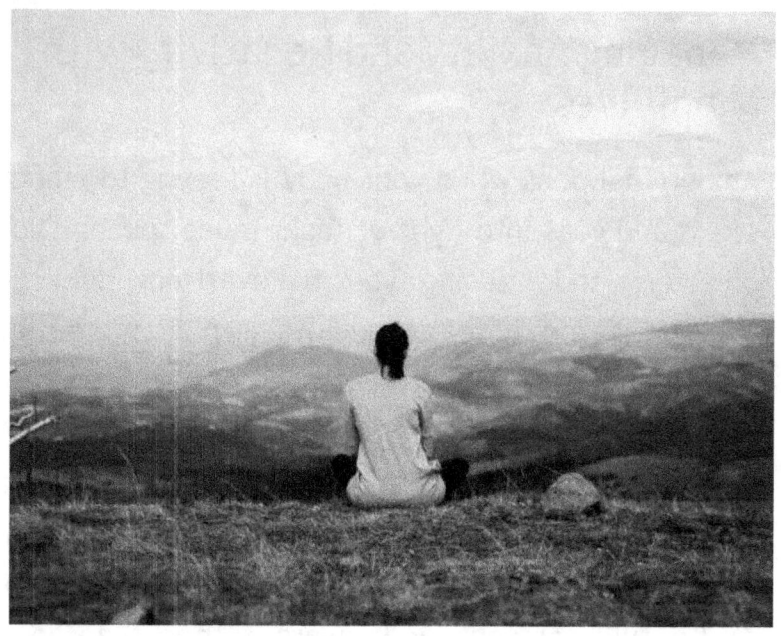

Mindfulness Techniques

Try these mindfulness techniques to help you navigate daily life with gentle and peaceful energy. Practicing these regularly is the key to success, so incorporate these techniques into your routine to build positive habits that will become second nature.

- **Body scan meditation:** Sit comfortably, close your eyes, and mentally scan your body from the tips of your toes to the top of your head, slowly, one limb at a time. This will help you notice and release the tension and stress you are holding in your body and help develop your awareness of your body without judgment. Release any tension you are holding on an exhale while consciously relaxing the muscle.

- **Grounding techniques** anchor you in the moment and bring you focus and clarity of thought.

- **Breath awareness** practices help calm your nervous system and reduce anxiety. Pay attention to your breathing and control the airflow with steady, counted inhalations and smooth exhalations. Feel the air fill your lungs and travel around your body, blowing away the anxiety.

- **Nonjudgmental observation** means observing your negative thoughts about your body image without judging or emotionally attaching to them. By being an impartial observer of the thoughts, you don't allow them to rule you. Labeling the negative thoughts as "judgments" will help you acknowledge them while recognizing their negativity so you can distance yourself from their impact.

- **Mindful eating**: Sit down to eat without distractions, and pay attention to what and how you are eating. Take your time, savor every bite, enjoy tastes, notice textures, and afterward, feel how your body responds to the nourishment.
- **Noticing triggers** will help you anticipate situations and thoughts that can negatively impact your recovery. Be mindful of your triggers and address them as soon as possible.
- **Cultivate gratitude** by focusing on the things you appreciate about your body and your life—this will shift you into a positive mindset!
- **Accept your emotions,** and don't try to fight or subdue them. Feel them, allow them to pass, and permit yourself to feel however you do in the moment.

Self-Awareness for Healing

Improving your self-awareness is another way you can support your mental health. There are two components of self-awareness: internal and external. Internal self-awareness is knowing your values, aspirations, emotions, behavior, strengths, and weaknesses. By knowing these things about yourself, you are able to identify your behavior patterns and weaknesses that can have a negative impact on your mental health and healing journey and develop coping mechanisms to prevent them from throwing you off track.

External self-awareness is understanding how other people perceive you based on the factors of internal self-awareness. Having good external self-awareness will help you be empathetic toward others and understand why they may react to or perceive you in a certain way—this will enable you to not dwell on the opinions of others and stop you from overanalyzing their comments and behavior.

Strong self-awareness has a powerful effect on your life in many ways and can help you take ownership of your body and mind. It will help you identify your triggers, recognize negative patterns of thought and behavior, and regulate your emotions so that you can make healthier choices and responses. Self-awareness will also encourage you to challenge and replace self-limiting and self-judging beliefs with positive and empowering thinking instead. Empowerment builds a sense of autonomy and control, which is crucial to your healing journey.

Stress reduction is another benefit of self-awareness since you'll be better equipped to manage stress and employ healthy coping mechanisms, as is an improved ability to make mindful decisions that prioritize your mental health and recovery. People with a strong sense of self-awareness often develop and maintain healthier relationships based on equality and empathy, which also means they find it easier to seek help, knowing that if they reach out for support, they will find it. Their relationships are built on kindness and patience on both sides, allowing them to be more at ease with themselves and more open and trusting with others. Finally, self-awareness also plays an essential role in recognizing the incredible growth and progress you undergo throughout your healing journey. Celebrating small victories and milestones on your journey will increase your self-awareness and also your sense of personal achievement in this challenging time.

Step 3 Activity: Guided Self-Compassion Exercises

Choose one of these three self-guided exercises to try today, depending on what you feel you need most. Each aims to open you up to self-compassion and bring positivity and tenderness into difficult or negative moments. You can do them anywhere, anytime, and whenever you need them.

Self-Compassion Stress Reliever

Sit comfortably and quietly, close your eyes, and call to mind a situation, thought, or feeling that is causing you stress or anxiety. Feel where the stress of it sits in your body. It may feel tight and tense or as though it is throbbing, aching, or painful. Find it and focus on it.

Say to yourself, "This is a moment of suffering and stress. It hurts."

Then say, "Suffering and stress are part of life. Everyone struggles. I am not alone."

Now, press your hand gently on the place where you feel your stress sitting. You can rub it tenderly or just let the palm of your hand bring warmth to it.

Say to yourself, "I give myself love and compassion and accept myself as I am. I am strong and capable and will get through this moment." Say whatever you most need to hear.

Breathe into the hand deeply until the tension dissipates and you are ready to open your eyes.

Self-Comforting Touch

This exercise will help you find a way to support and comfort yourself through a simple touch action. Think of it like cuddling yourself—hugging helps calm nerves and makes you feel safe, like a baby in its mother's arms. The touch of a gentle hand on your skin activates positive chemicals that are soothing.

Explore your body and find a spot and action that feels comforting to touch and brings you a sense of calmness. It could be:

- your chest over your heart
- a hand on your cheek
- giving yourself a hug and stroking your arms
- a hand on your stomach
- holding your own hand
- cupping your face in your hands
- stroking your own hair
- rubbing your temples or forehead in circles

When you feel stressed or anxious, stop what you're doing and place your hand on your comfort spot. Breathe deeply into that spot as you perform your soothing action, and keep going until you feel comforted and ready to carry on with your day.

Challenging Critical Self-Talk

You can either write your way through this exercise, speak aloud, or think silently, whatever works best for you or the circumstances.

Notice when you are being self-critical. It may be a little voice in your head that appears out of nowhere and makes you feel bad about yourself or something you have done, like eating junk food. Hear what it says, the tone it says it in, and make sure you can identify it clearly. It might say things like, "You're disgusting," or "You make me sick."

When you hear it, work to soften its blow by offering it compassion and understanding. Say to it, "I know you're only saying that because you're afraid and worried about me, but it hurts me."

Now, invite your self-compassionate voice to take its place. How do you need to be spoken to in this moment to bring positivity and understanding? Try saying, "I know you're feeling sad and stressed, and that's why you did what you did. You hoped it would make things better, but it didn't. You don't feel good in your body right now, and that's okay. What will make you feel happy right now?"

Let this kind inner voice bring you comfort and tenderness in a tough moment, and allow it to lead you toward taking positive action that makes you feel better.

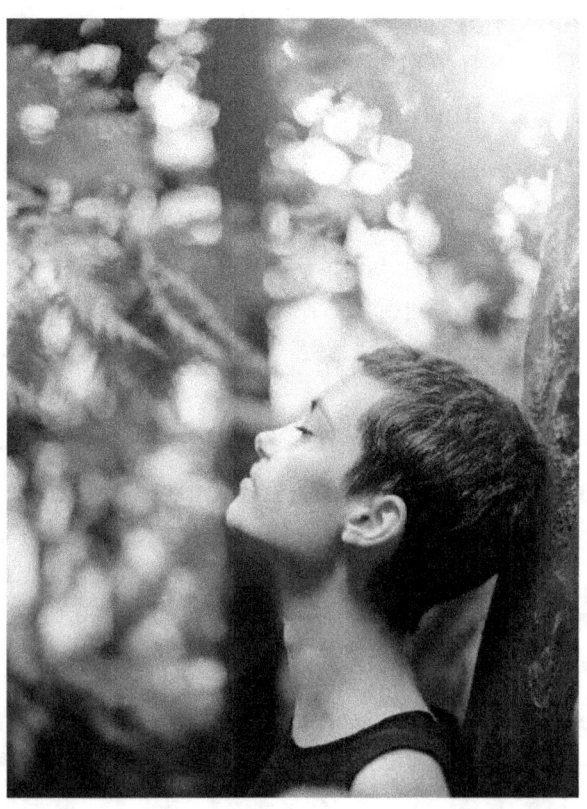

Challenging that inner self-critical voice is one step toward unraveling negative and harmful self-talk that has trapped you in an unhealthy body image mindset for so long. Negative self-talk has a potent and painful hold on your emotions and self-image, and in the next chapter, we'll explore some ways to overcome it.

Chapter 4
Step 4 - Unraveling Negative Thought Patterns

For most people, the majority of thoughts they have in a day are negative: about money, goals, chores, people, and themselves. It can be hard to see the positives in life when times are tough, and the negative aspects have the most significant impact. Negative thoughts have a domino effect on your mood, health, behavior, and perspective on life. For people with body dysmorphia, these effects can have long-term consequences and make recovery exceptionally difficult. To heal, you'll need to break out of negative thought patterns and open up your body and mind to the powerful energy of positive thinking.

The Connection Between Thoughts, Emotions, and Behavior

A deep and unique connection exists between your thoughts, emotions, and behavior. They each have a strong influence over each other, and each will drive your actions and responses throughout the day. Your thoughts and beliefs about situations and events can trigger an emotional response, such as fear, anxiety, or joy, and these feelings, in turn, will influence how your body reacts and how you behave in that situation. Your emotions shape your thoughts and how you perceive the world, coloring how you interpret events and actions, which can distort your thinking and behavior. Thought and belief can be a driving force of behavior for good and bad. Believing you are capable of achieving something makes you more likely to succeed because you approach it with the confidence and determination to succeed. Conversely, if you think negatively about yourself, your behavior will reflect that, leading to avoidant behavior or a lack of effort. Positive and rewarding behavior promotes healthy and happy emotions and encourages you to keep pursuing that behavior, whereas negative behaviors can increase feelings of guilt, shame, and sadness.

Understanding and adapting this complex network of cause and effect, this continuous cycle of influence will be an essential part of your recovery journey. The idea that behavior, thought, and feeling are intrinsically linked is the core principle of cognitive behavioral therapy (CBT). CBT is not only one of the most effective forms of treatment for body dysmorphia and eating disorders, but it is effective for a wide range of associated mental health issues as well.

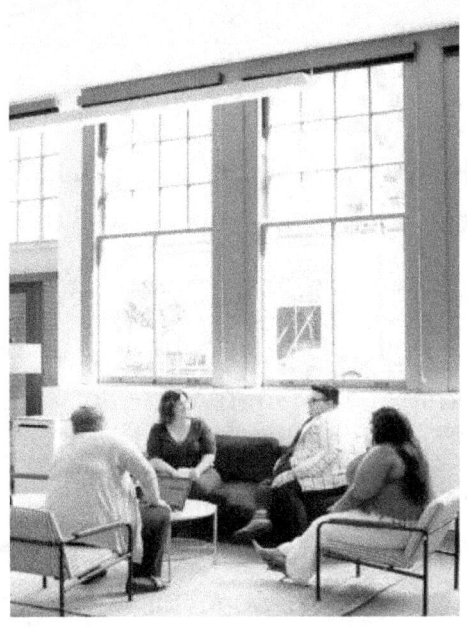

Cognitive Behavioral Therapy

What is Cognitive Behavioral Therapy?

CBT is a widely used form of psychotherapy that concentrates on changing your mindset, thought patterns, and behavior, to help relieve mental health symptoms. Working with a psychotherapist, you will practice identifying, challenging, and changing the negative thoughts that come with your body dysmorphia or eating disorder so you can adapt to a more positive mindset and behaviors in the future. CBT isn't just talking about your feelings; it is a structured and personalized approach to mental health therapy full of techniques and practices you will develop with your psychotherapist over time.

CBT focuses on helping you form new and positive habits and ways of approaching your body image issues so that you can reduce and manage your stress and anxiety, develop effective coping mechanisms, and shift your thinking to a more balanced and emotionally healthy outlook. There are several benefits to cognitive behavioral therapy. Such a short-term treatment (usually up to 20 sessions) can have long-term results; it is a flexible treatment that offers group, one-on-one, or solo formats, making it a great alternative to medicine. The skills you learn through CBT will become a vital part of your life and may continue to shape and inform your thinking and behavior for years. These skills impact many areas of your life, not just your body image and mental health but also your problem-solving, time management, communication, and social skills.

So, how does CBT work?

Cognitive Behavioral Therapy Techniques to Combat Negative Thinking

CBT aims to change your negative thinking into positive thinking through a variety of techniques and exercises that require you to take an active part in your recovery. While you may talk about your past and any trauma with your therapist, the focus will be much more on your present situation and health and on setting practices in place to build a better future for you.

Negative thinking manifests in many forms, including catastrophizing, thinking in black and white, overgeneralizing, and focusing on the negatives. These negative thought patterns may appear as a mean voice in your head saying all the things you fear most, or they may arise as overwhelming emotions of anger, fear, and sadness when triggered by a stimulus or situation. Negative thoughts can stem from your core beliefs, which are ingrained in you through your childhood experiences and are at the center of how you see yourself. They can also come from dysfunctional and irrational assumptions you've held onto based on negative comments or experiences you've had and also from habitual or automatic negative thoughts that appear briefly and without warning in response to a trigger. Below are some CBT techniques therapists use to help to reframe negative thoughts.

- **Cognitive restructuring** consists of identifying negative or irrational thought patterns and beliefs and using evidence and rational or positive thoughts to challenge and replace their validity.
- **Thought records** are worksheets that help you identify negative thoughts and emotions and their associated situations or triggers. The worksheet will encourage you to give evidence for and against the thoughts to give you a clearer perspective and a more balanced mindset.

- **Cognitive reframing** helps you to change how you interpret and view situations, putting them in a positive or realistic light rather than a negative one so you can limit the impact of negative thoughts.

- **Decatastrophizing:** Catastrophizing is a typical negative thought pattern where you habitually believe that the worst will happen, no matter how irrational or unlikely that is— this can provoke intense anxiety and fear and prevent you from taking risks or pushing your boundaries. Decatastrophizing involves asking yourself questions that interrupt catastrophic thinking and make you assess the reality of the situation so you can understand if you are really in danger of what you're worried about.

- **Mindfulness-based cognitive therapy** combines mindfulness practices with CBT techniques to encourage you to observe your thoughts and emotions without judgment and allow them to pass without holding on to them—this helps you break out of negative thought patterns.

- **Behavioral activation:** By building a positive mindset and outlook through engaging in activities you enjoy or find fulfilling, you'll counteract negative thoughts and emotions.

- **Graded exposure** helps you challenge your fears and triggers by gradually and in a controlled way exposing you to them. This also helps to reduce avoidance and expand your comfort zone.
- **Coping cards:** carry positive affirmations and coping statements, so you have them on hand to remind you of healthier coping responses.
- **Identifying core beliefs**: Challenging and understanding your deep-rooted core beliefs about yourself can help you reevaluate and address your behavior and negative thought patterns.

Journaling and Cognitive Reframing Exercises

Journaling is an integral part of CBT. It is a potent tool for self-compassion, self-awareness, reflection, and personal growth, and it also helps you to track your progress and recognize patterns of thought and behavior throughout your healing journey. Specific, CBT-based prompts help you dig deep into your thoughts, emotions, and behavior to bring you clarity and help you make positive changes in your life. CBT journal prompts should be very specific and tailored to your needs and goals. Your therapist will assign prompts that target your unique needs, the challenges you face, and the areas of your life you need to address in order to enjoy a successful recovery. As part of your CBT journey, journaling will become part of your daily routine.

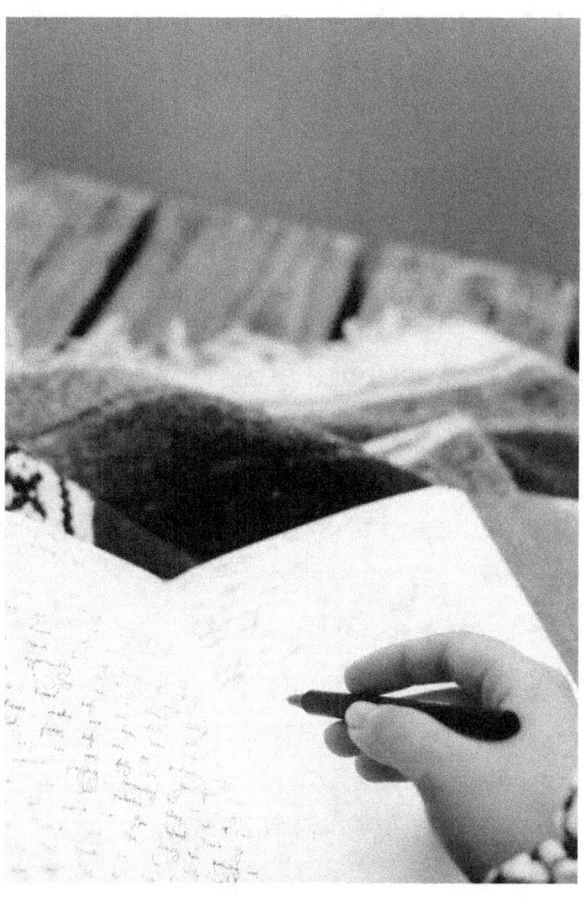

Step 4 Activity: Positive Journaling

Get yourself a notebook and pen, and try these journal prompts to get you started. Answer honestly and be open to your feelings without judgment—this is for your eyes only.

1. Reflect on a recent situation that triggered a strong emotion in you, such as anxiety, fear, or anger. Describe what happened and what thoughts went through your mind at the time. Can you recognize any cognitive distortions in your response to the situation?

2. Pick a persistent negative thought or belief that you experience often. What evidence supports this belief? What evidence contradicts it? Reframe the thought to be more balanced and realistic based on the evidence.

3. Reflect on a situation in which your emotions and thoughts influenced your behavior. What were the consequences of your reaction? How would you respond differently if it happened again?

4. Describe a recent challenge you faced. How did you overcome it? What coping

techniques did you use? What would you do differently next time?

5. Reflect on a recent interaction that you found difficult. What thoughts and feelings were present at the time? How did these thoughts and feelings influence your behavior?

6. What negative thoughts have you experienced today? How did they make you feel? How did you behave because of them? What evidence is there to contradict these thoughts? What is a more positive, rational, or balanced perspective you could take instead?

7. Reflect on a positive change you have made recently, a positive experience you have had, or something positive you have accomplished. How did it change your behavior and outlook? What thoughts went through your head?

Prompts like these force you to take the time to dig into your psyche. They can be overwhelming and challenging to answer initially, but commit to your journaling practice, and you'll find it easier to reflect with compassion and understanding over time.

Your mind is only one half of the puzzle in your journey back to health. As we'll discover in the next chapter, your body needs care and attention, too, and neither body nor mind can thrive without nourishment.

Chapter 5
Step 5 - Nourishing Your Body and Mind

Body dysmorphia and eating disorders have enormous negative impacts on physical health, and while no two bodies are the same, they all need the same essential care: nourishment and exercise. Many eating disorders and body image issues arise from trying to attain unnatural and impossible beauty standards. A healthy body does not mean a skinny one or one you see in movies or on TV—it means a body that is strong and can support you through your daily life and the demands and challenges you face. You need to accept the limitations of your body and your body type and embrace your body as it is while finding ways to support it and give it what it needs so that it can carry you through the challenges and adventures of life.

The Physical/Mental Health Connection

Mental and physical health are intricately connected, and body dysmorphia and eating disorders heavily impact both. Suppose your mind is in a constant state of anxiety, fear, and negativity. In that case, your body responds by going into survival mode, which puts a lot of pressure on your organs, muscles, and nervous system and is exhausting—the body isn't supposed to exist in a state of flight-or-fight for long periods of time. When eating disorders take hold, the body and mind suffer in many ways.

Physical conditions, like chronic illness, pain, disabilities, and long-term injuries, often cause psychological distress, anxiety, and depression, which directly impacts mental well-being and encourages a negative mindset. Pain, illness, and injury often severely impact appetite and your ability to exercise, causing fluctuations in weight, which can exacerbate body image issues. Chronic inflammation—a common result of injury, surgery, disease, or a joint disorder—can be linked to depression and other mental health disorders, making your body a very unpleasant place to inhabit, which also aggravates body dysmorphia. Medications to treat physical conditions and pain can have side effects that influence your mental health and mood, so be sure to check with your doctor about the role this may play in your recovery. Maintaining good physical health enhances your resilience to illness and injury. Also, it improves your ability to heal, boosting recovery time and lessening the chance of developing long-term disorders and issues, which in turn have a detrimental impact on mental health.

Your hormones play a vital role in your mental and physical health: Your endocrine system is directly linked to your brain's neurotransmitters, meaning hormonal imbalances—which are common in people with eating disorders—have a domino effect on mood and behavior, often leading to depression and increased anxiety. Similarly, your gut and brain are linked via the gut-brain axis, meaning your gut health, influenced mainly by your diet, directly affects your mood and mental health.

Physical health issues can cause stress, and some physical conditions also have underlying psychological causes, such as stress and anxiety. Stress can manifest in the body as headaches and migraines, gastrointestinal issues, and even psychogenic pain, which is pain without a physical cause. Finding effective coping techniques, like mindfulness and relaxation, to deal with psychological factors is an integral part of physical recovery.

Illness and injury—particularly long-term ones—can sometimes lead to social isolation and discrimination, which are both risk factors for mental health problems. People suffering from illness and injury can be afraid of being a burden or not feeling up to taking part in social activities because they get quickly tired or can't join in. When they isolate themselves, they are forced to sit with their negative thoughts and feelings without distraction or relief, which can lead to depression.

Mental health disorders such as anxiety and depression can be very exhausting but, at the same time, interfere with your ability to sleep properly. This means you often feel worn out and de-energized, making it very difficult to get up, exercise, or find the energy to cook, all leading to a weakened physical state, a poor diet, and a burnt-out brain. In this state, your body and mind both suffer greatly, so it is vital that you find ways to supercharge your energy levels so that your mental health doesn't drag you down. One way to do this is by ensuring you consume a healthy, balanced, and nutritional diet that can fuel and support you throughout the day, even on a bad one.

Establishing Healthy Eating Habits

A nutritional and balanced diet is a necessity for a healthy body and mind, but when you have an eating disorder or body dysmorphia, food can quickly become an "enemy." Forming a negative relationship with food in order to lose and control your weight has enormous repercussions on your health, weakening your body and triggering unhealthy associations and irrational perceptions of food. Rebuilding trust in food and a positive relationship with your diet is a crucial step in your recovery, and it begins with understanding why a healthy diet matters.

Nutritional Awareness

The nutritional value of what you are eating is incredibly important. While in recovery, you may struggle with portion sizes and regular eating, but if you can control the nutritional value of what you *do* eat, then you'll stay a step ahead. A small meal full of vitamins and minerals is better than nothing or too much with little nutritional value!

Your body needs specific essential nutrition, which it receives best from a varied and balanced diet that contains all of the food groups in the correct amounts. Each of the food groups contributes to your body's needs and functions, contributing essential macronutrients (carbohydrates, proteins, and fats) and micronutrients (vitamins and minerals). Poor nutrition has a massive impact on your physical and mental well-being, including:

- lower immunity, leading to more frequent illness and a longer recovery time
- low energy levels and fatigue
- weakened bones and muscle
- skin breakouts, hair loss, and brittle nails
- dental problems
- more likely to binge eat to sate cravings
- increased risk of developing severe health problems like heart disease, diabetes, and some cancers
- inability to focus and problems with memory
- disrupted sleep
- mood swings and increased depression

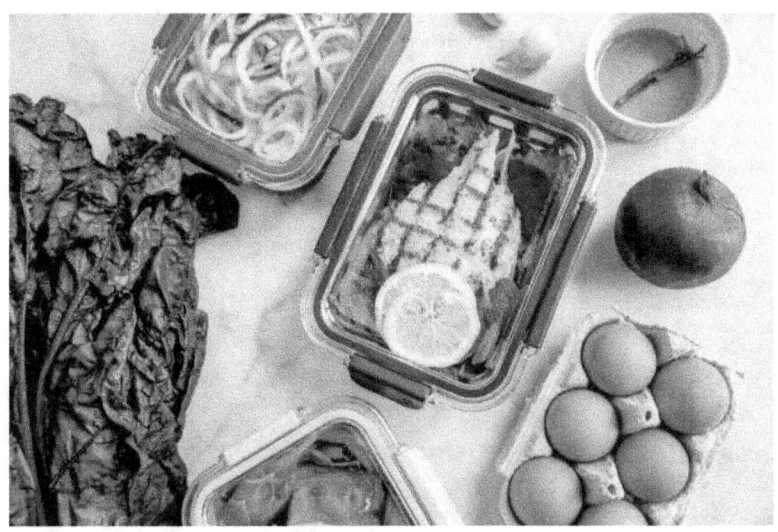

Healthy Eating Habits

It's easy to say, "I'll start to eat better," but building healthy eating habits while you are recovering from an eating disorder or living with body dysmorphia can feel impossible. The guilt and shame you might feel around food can make you extremely anxious when approaching your diet and can lead you to make poor nutritional choices. Here are some great habits to build into your daily life to improve your relationship with food and get you on track to a healthier lifestyle.

- **Eat a balanced diet** of various foods from each food group. Make your meals colorful with delicious fruits and vegetables, prioritize whole grains over refined grains, and incorporate healthy fats and lean proteins (such as poultry and fish) into your diet.

- **Portion control** is an excellent tool for limiting your eating, whether to control overeating or encourage you to eat more. Use smaller plates and bowls to lower your portion size, or set yourself the goal of finishing a whole plate of food to increase your portions.

- **Mindful eating** means paying attention to what you are eating in the moment and noticing your hunger and fullness cues. When you eat, savor your food and flavors, limit distractions, and allow yourself to enjoy giving your body what it needs.

- **Plan and prepare meals** in advance so that you know what you will be eating and can take the time to ensure you have nutritional meals readily available. It also helps you to control what you are eating, your cooking methods, and your portion sizes.

- **Read food labels** to comprehend the nutritional content of what you are eating. Look for products that are lower in sugar, sodium, and unhealthy fats.
- **Hydrate!** Water is essential for optimal body functioning and also plays a part in regulating appetite and optimizing nutrient absorption. Aim to drink a glass of water every hour—you can even set a reminder on your phone for it!
- **Limit processed and high-sugar foods:** These foods have little nutritional value, and their chemicals and sugar can encourage binge eating and other negative eating habits. Always choose whole or natural foods instead.
- **Enjoy healthy snacks** such as nuts, seeds, fruit, yogurt, and whole grain cereals to curb cravings for unhealthy snacks between meals.
- **Eating slowly** helps with digestion and nutrient intake, so take your time to eat so that you don't feel bloated and will feel full for longer.
- **Listen to your body**; it will tell you how it is feeling, when it is hungry or not, and if certain foods aren't good for it. Allergies

and intolerances play a considerable part in your diet, so make sure you get help for them and work your diet around them.

- **Consult a dietician:** They can give you guidance on building a better diet, help you reach your health goals, and address your concerns.

Meal Planning

Meal planning will be a very useful tool in your recovery journey, even if you aren't diagnosed with an eating disorder. When you plan and prepare meals in advance, you ensure you get the nutrients you need to keep your body strong and feeling good. You can exercise more control over your diet, so there's no fear of ingesting something unexpected that may make you feel bad later. It also removes the need to think about your next meal, so you aren't dwelling on food constantly. Sticking to a meal plan encourages good eating habits, like keeping regular meal times and setting suitable portion sizes. Knowing ahead of time what you will be eating on any given day takes the anxiety of choice away and also helps you avoid snacking or buying junk food to quell a craving.

Work with a registered dietician or your recovery team to ensure you tailor your diet to your needs. If you are cooking or meal planning for someone with body dysmorphia or an eating disorder, work with them in your planning and make sure they feel their needs are seen and accounted for—this will help give them a more positive perception of the meals rather than feel they have no choice.

Every day of your meal plan should account for breakfast, lunch, and dinner, plus a healthy and energizing afternoon snack. Three meals a day may initially sound excessive and intimidating, but **start small**. Your portions don't have to be huge. The important thing is that you are eating regularly and making sure your body has something to run on. Even if you aren't hungry, try not to skip a meal entirely—eating even a little is better than none at all!

Exercise for Your Mental Well-Being

Exercise has a powerful impact on your mental health and can be vital to recovery. It puts you in touch with your body and mind and helps you to feel supported, confident, and in control of your body, boosting your self-esteem and self-image. Exercise triggers the release of endorphins, a chemical that acts as a natural mood-lifter and reduces feelings of stress, anxiety, and depression. It also helps to balance the neurotransmitters in your brain that regulate mood—serotonin and dopamine—so your mood doesn't fluctuate so much, and you feel more emotionally stable. The reduction of stress is another benefit of exercise. When you exercise, your energy focuses on the physical work required, relieving the pressure on your mind, distracting you from negative thoughts, and allowing you to take a much-needed break from your anxieties. With regular exercise, the symptoms of depression and anxiety can reduce as your brain gets more time off and your confidence and comfort in your body increase. Stress reduction also comes from an increased ability to *deal* with stress. Exercise can help you build your resilience, and it is a positive and healthy coping mechanism for life's emotional and practical challenges. Exercise has also been proven to significantly improve brain function, enhancing memory and concentration.

Engaging in team sports and group exercise, such as a yoga class, helps you build connections, prevents feelings of isolation and loneliness, and encourages you to open up. Having fun exercising with other people to distract you from your body and your negative thoughts makes exercise more manageable and makes you more likely to stick with it. They can also help you attain your fitness goals, which, big or small, will give you a wonderful sense of achievement and satisfaction and remind you that you and your body are capable of anything.

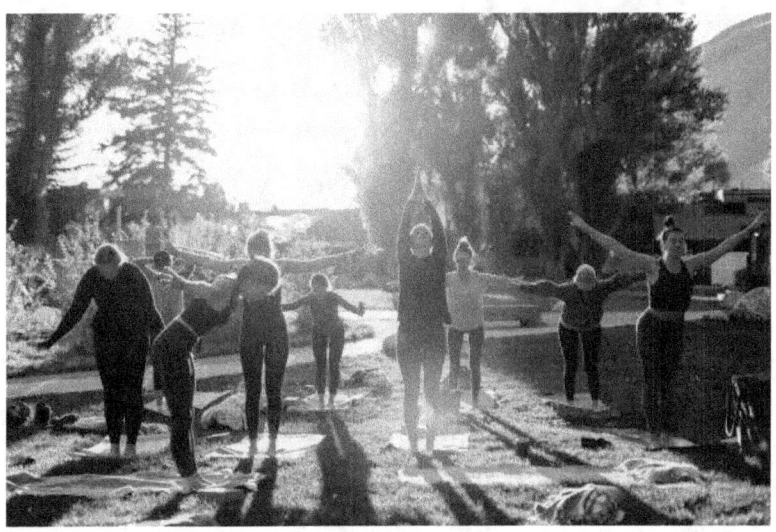

Get Moving!

Maintaining a consistent exercise routine will give your life structure and a sense of control, but sticking to a routine can be most difficult, especially on a bad day when your negative thoughts are bringing you down and draining your energy. You mustn't let them stop you from making progress, so here are a few tips to make exercise easier, more manageable, and more fun for you.

- **Start slow and low:** Your body needs time to build up strength and stamina, so starting with intense cardio workouts and heavy weights will be overwhelming and painful, and you'll be more likely to injure yourself. Ease your body into exercise with gentle warm-ups and exercise that is appropriate for your level of fitness. Work your way up to longer exercise sessions and more weekly exercise over time.
- **Break it up:** You don't have to cram all your weekly exercise into one session. Instead, split it into manageable sessions of up to 30 minutes a day or even less if you have a busy schedule. Even ten minutes of yoga at your desk is better than doing nothing at all.
- **Get creative!** Exercise doesn't have to be repetitive and mindless—choose activities that you enjoy and change things up if they get dull. Fill your routine with various options like swimming, dance classes, cycling, and Pilates to keep you engaged and excited to exercise.

- **Listen to your body**; it will tell you if something isn't working for you and if something is. Sharp pain, shortness of breath, nausea, and dizziness are all signs that you need to stop and rest. Pushing yourself to the point of collapse is never a good idea—exercise should make you feel energized and exhilarated!

- **Stay flexible:** Not physically, although yoga can help with that, but be flexible with your routine. Some days, your body will not be up to exercising, and that's okay. Give yourself a break and return refreshed and ready to pick up where you left off.

- **Ignore your mirror!** It can take time for the results of your hard work to show on your body, so don't expect miracles overnight. Instead, focus your attention inward and enjoy the journey for yourself.

Step 5 Activity: Mindful Eating Practice

Your activity for this step is to practice mindful eating during one meal every day. As you eat, pay attention to your food's tastes, textures, and sensations, take your time to eat, and spend the whole meal exploring your food rather than judging it. Afterward, write down the following:

- how the experience made you feel while you were doing it
- how you feel after the meal
- what you feared or what worried you before the meal
- how those fears sit now that you have eaten
- three positive things about the meal, e.g., how it will nourish your body or how it tasted

Keep up this practice for at least a week and see how your mealtime mindset shifts.

Your health is one of the most important things in your life, and taking care of yourself mentally and physically is a huge task—one made difficult by triggering situations that can set your progress back and send you spiraling. In the next chapter, we'll look at how to identify and cope with these triggers so that you can keep moving forward in your recovery journey.

Chapter 6
Step 6 - Identifying and Coping With Triggers

Life doesn't come with trigger warnings. Every time you step out of your door or look at your phone, you open yourself up to potential triggers. You simply can't avoid them—if you tried to, you'd spend your whole life hiding, and that's no life at all! Instead, you must find ways to face your triggers, understand them, and overcome them using coping techniques and self-awareness. Everyone has different triggers, and you might not know yours until they appear, which is why they are such a scary concept. Luckily, there are healthy and positive ways to protect yourself.

What Are Triggers?

Triggers are stimuli that evoke a traumatic memory and cause a behavioral and emotional response in you. Triggers can appear as sounds, sensations, smells, words, times, and even people—anything that causes a memory of trauma to resurface unexpectedly and force you to relive that event. The trigger activates a response in you, often as a heightened negative emotion like fear or anger, and in many cases of mental health, the trigger provokes and worsens the symptoms of your condition. Triggers are a frightening prospect because they can appear out of nowhere and can feel very isolating and exposing.

Body Image Triggers

There are a number of common triggers for body dysmorphia and body image issues, many of which you encounter multiple times a day, which makes them hard to avoid. Social media and the influence of film and TV often promote and idealize unrealistic body images, which can trigger feelings of inadequacy and fuel body dysmorphia. It also fuels comparisons, as you compare your body to those you see in the media—this leads to dissatisfaction and anxiety. The prevalence of the media and social media in our lives makes this one of the most common triggers you will encounter. The pressure to conform to society and the media's body image standards through the way you dress is another trigger. Shopping for clothes can be an overwhelming and anxiety-ridden experience as clothes are often made for certain idealized body types, and trends usually cater to whatever body type is currently "in."

One of the primary triggers for body image issues is trauma. Traumatic experiences related to your body, appearance, or weight contribute heavily to body dysmorphia and anxiety, and reactions to these triggers can be extreme and frightening. While avoiding situations that may trigger traumatic memories can help, avoidant behavior can reinforce negative thought patterns and further trigger your body image anxiety.

Negative comments and criticism about your appearance are more often a fear than a reality, but occasionally, someone will say something that triggers you. Family, friends, and peers can say things without meaning to trigger your dysmorphia, or they may even believe they are paying you a compliment. People with body dysmorphia and the anxiety that accompanies it are more emotionally sensitive to perceived criticism and negative comments and will often overanalyze comments and take them very deeply to heart. Any situation that puts you in the spotlight, like performing, participating in sports, or even giving a presentation, can be triggering, as it opens you up to perceived judgments and puts you and your body on display.

Feeling a lack of control over your life can spark anxiety and increase your body image distress. Personal stressors, like work, relationships, and financial stress, can be particularly triggering. They can make you feel very intense emotions and put you under a lot of pressure, which can lead you to focus on negatives and apply that pressure to your body or try to exercise more control of your body when your personal stressors make you feel out of control.

Natural and unavoidable changes in your body are also common triggers. Pregnancy, motherhood, puberty, illness, aging, and weight fluctuations are all common triggers for people with body dysmorphia, as there is very little you can do about them. Your body changes in ways that you cannot control, and this can be very scary, making you feel out of control and even betrayed by your body. Accepting these changes is the work of a lifetime, and you'll find you need to relearn how to love your body over and over again in order to live the happy and fulfilling life you deserve.

Identifying Your Triggers

Everyone responds differently to their triggers; sometimes, your response may seem irrational and disproportionate to outsiders. That's okay! Your triggers and mental health are your business, and how you respond is personal to you. Coping with and identifying your triggers will help you anticipate them and regulate your reaction to them. Here are some methods of identifying and understanding your triggers:

- **Practice self-awareness** by paying attention to your emotions in the moment and noticing their intensity. Are they positive or negative emotions? When you have a strong emotional reaction to something, take the time to process it.
- **Reflect on your past experiences** and times when you have had strong emotional reactions. Ask yourself the following questions:

- ○ What were the common factors in these situations?
- ○ Were there any specific people, events, or circumstances that triggered you in these moments?
- ○ How did you handle yourself in these moments?
- ○ Were you self-compassionate, or did you allow negativity to rule your reaction?
- ○ What would you do differently?

- **Journaling** is a very effective method of identifying and tracking your triggers. By writing about your feelings and experiences regularly, you can start to see patterns in behavior and the recurring themes, experiences, and emotions that provoke an emotional reaction.
- **Mindfulness and meditation** will enhance your self-awareness and train you to sit with your feelings without judgment, enabling you to explore the reasons behind them.
- **Talk to others.** Discuss emotional experiences with friends, family, or your therapist. An outside perspective may help you see situations differently and help you

identify triggers you didn't pick up on at the time.

- **Notice physical cues.** Emotional triggers can manifest as a physical response, such as rapid heartbeat, high blood pressure, headaches, exhaustion, nausea, and stomach problems.
- **Identify common themes** in your behavior and thought patterns. You might notice that when you're stressed or have an impending deadline, you tend to be more critical of yourself or experience anxiety more intensely.
- **Monitor your thoughts** during emotionally charged situations—certain thoughts and beliefs may provoke your responses.
- **Use trigger lists.** You'll find them online, and they list common triggers to help you identify yours. Trigger lists categorize triggers into areas of life, like relationships or work, which can enable you to narrow down particular areas you find difficult.

Be patient with yourself throughout your trigger explorations. This is a difficult part of your recovery, filled with reflections on past events and a heightened awareness of the present.

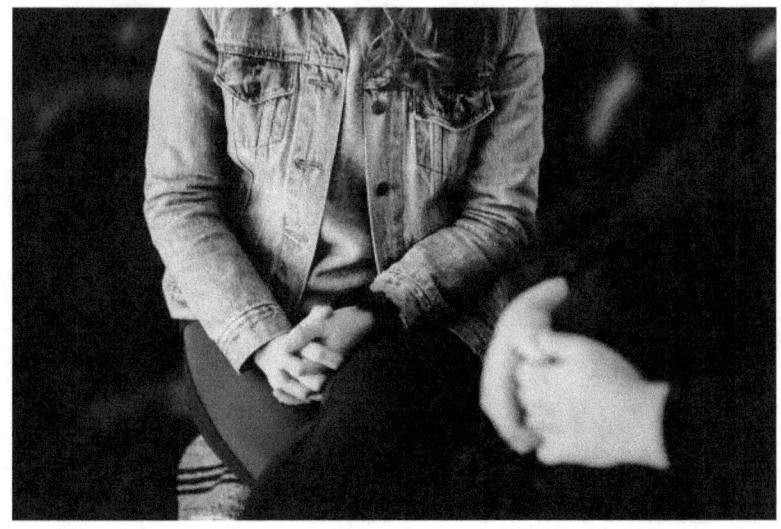

Coping Strategies

You're going to need some coping strategies at the ready for when things trigger you. Triggers will set off an emotional reaction that, if unchecked, can send you spiraling toward unhealthy coping mechanisms or lead to volatile behavior that can damage your relationships. It can cause you unnecessary suffering, leaving you overwhelmed with fear and sadness, which damages your mental health and can hold you back from reaching out to others and exploring new life experiences.

Avoidant behavior is a common coping mechanism but an ineffective one in the long term. Avoiding a trigger—such as a social event or a meal—makes you feel better and safer in the moment, but the emotion will return soon and stronger, so you'll need to adopt more—and often more extreme—avoidant behaviors in order to cope. The more you need to avoid, the more anxious you'll get, and the feelings will compound and get more invasive and intense. Instead of avoiding, you must face your emotions and triggers and learn to regulate your emotional reactions.

Emotional self-regulation is a learned skill that will be very useful for dealing with triggering situations. It will help you filter and control your reactions and allow you to process your emotions with more understanding and self-compassion. Emotional regulation involves dialing down the intensity of an emotion, not suppressing or avoiding it so that you can control how you express emotion. You will still feel the emotion, but instead of being consumed by it, you take the time to acknowledge and validate it, interpret what the emotion is telling you, and use that knowledge to respond. Regulation buys you time to respond appropriately to a trigger rather than reacting on instinct out of fear, anxiety, or pain.

Four Emotional Regulation Techniques

Use these four simple but effective techniques for emotional regulation to help you overcome your triggers and improve your mental well-being.

Pause and Make Space

When emotions are triggered, they come out of nowhere fast and intense. It can feel like hurtling headfirst into a black hole, so the best thing you can do is give yourself time and space to process. Take a deep breath, then another. Let the moment happen, and provide it with room to settle. Slow down the time between the trigger and your emotional response. Stay present.

Tune In to Your Body and Mind

Triggers can set off a physical reaction such as an increased heart rate, trouble breathing, sweating, shaking, teeth grinding, sudden tension, and an urge to cry or scream. These reactions are symptoms of the emotional turmoil within and your body becoming unbalanced and entering survival mode. Focus on what you are feeling physically, zone in on where your body is reacting, and try to relax that area. You can imagine the area is glowing red, and as you relax, the glow turns blue, then white when calm is restored. This will help to distract your mind and intensify the emotions you're feeling.

Name What You Feel

Emotions can be overwhelming in the moment, but take a pause to name what you are feeling. Break the emotions down to their simplest state, such as anger, fear, or resentment. Next, identify what is making you feel that emotion. What are you angry about? What are you afraid will happen? Naming your emotions helps to simplify them and make them less intimidating.

If you feel up to it, or if you need support, you can explain your reaction to someone more clearly by naming your emotions. Instead of lashing out, say, "I feel angry because..." and help them to understand. They'll be more likely to show you compassion and support and may even be able to help you in similar situations in the future.

Promote Positivity

You can quickly see only the negatives in a situation when triggered, and humans tend to catastrophize in a crisis. Still, if you take a moment to find positive things around you or in your life, the negatives won't seem so terrible. In any triggering situation, or even just when you're having a bad day, notice the positive things around you, things that make you feel grateful and content, and things you find interesting or fun. Negative feelings weigh heavy on you, but positive ones can lift you up and boost your resilience and energy.

Positive self-talk, or reframing, is also a great coping technique in triggering times. Even if you feel terrible, be kind and compassionate to yourself with soothing and supportive words that strengthen your self-belief and calm your mind.

Step 6 Activity: Trigger Journal

For a week, keep a journal tracking your triggers. Make a note of events, situations, conversations, or even social media posts that trigger your negative body image thoughts and anxieties. Then, ask yourself these questions:

- How did you feel when triggered?
- How did you cope in the moment?
- What was the effect of the trigger? Were there any physical effects?
- What did the negative voice in your head say? How could you reword it to be kinder?
- Was there someone you could have turned to for support? Did you?

Using the coping strategies above, find healthy ways to work around the triggers.

While this chapter has been tough, full of complex ideas and self-searching, there's a bright light ahead in the next chapter, where we'll explore the wonderful world of body positivity and how learning to respect and appreciate your body will boost your recovery and help you learn to love yourself again.

Chapter 7
Step 7 - Embracing Body Acceptance and Positivity

It is rare to find someone who is happy with their body. Everyone has something about themselves that bugs them; everyone wants to improve their body or enhance a feature in order to meet an idealized image they have of themselves. For most people, these are fleeting thoughts that quickly fade away in the face of life's challenges and joys, but for those with body dysmorphia, these thoughts and self-perceptions rule the whole day and almost every decision you make. Learning to love and accept the body you have is a vital step in your recovery and will allow you to lead a fulfilled and happy life without the constant cloud of negativity and judgment that your condition brings. Trying to change your body using the extreme methods often associated with eating disorders and body dysmorphia not only damages your body but also alienates you from it, meaning it is harder for you to understand and accept yourself and see yourself for who you really are. Practicing body positivity will help you reconnect with yourself and your body and give you a healthier perception of the human body.

The Power of Body Positivity

What is Body Positivity?

Body positivity is a social movement that aims to boost self-esteem and mental well-being by promoting love and acceptance of the human body in all its shapes, sizes, skin tones, and genders. Aiming to promote self-acceptance, reduce the stigma associated with weight, and encourage people to celebrate their bodies, body positivity challenges society and the media's unrealistic and unattainable beauty standards. It also advocates for a more diverse representation of bodies in the media, confronting stereotypical depictions of race, gender, and certain body types and working to relieve the burden of conformity. By improving your relationship with your body through body positivity, you foster respect for your body and gain a healthier perspective on body image. Body positivity also encourages a healthier relationship with food and exercise. Instead of strict diets and excessive exercise, you are encouraged to listen to your body's needs and eat and exercise however makes you happy. While celebrating individuality is central to body positivity, it has also created a vast and supportive community with shared goals and experiences where you can be yourself without judgment or ridicule.

Body positivity plays an essential role in improving mental health, predominantly for those who struggle with body dysmorphia and eating disorders, helping you to feel more confident and at ease in your body, encouraging self-compassion, and promoting a positive view of self-worth, demonstrating that your body doesn't signify your value. With these principles, you can live a less anxious, happier, and more fulfilling life.

Challenging Beauty Standards

One of the key aims of body positivity is to challenge the unrealistic beauty standards set by society, fashion, and the media. You are exposed to and confronted by these beauty standards all day on screens, in advertisements, in songs, and in magazines. Social media is particularly problematic, a realm of cyberbullying, fad diets, and beauty trends that are more often than not heavily edited, unaffordable, and have no proven results. Social media doesn't allow for differences in body type and personal situation, and it is easy to buy into what you see working for someone else at the expense of your own health. Fashion is often designed for certain, idealized body types rather than for a broader range of types. Because of social media, there is even greater pressure than ever on people to dress with the trends and fit into societal ideals. All of these unattainable and unsustainable standards have conspired to create an unhealthy environment. When you don't see your own body represented in a positive way and respected by society and the media, it damages your self-esteem. It makes you feel invisible or unworthy of notice.

Body positivity will help you fight against these standards and encourage you to see past the lies, edits, and trends to recognize that everyone's body is different, and you have to do what is best for your body and mind. Trends and fads come and go, but your body is yours for life, and by respecting it for the fantastic job it does getting you through the day, you can see that what you wear and how your body looks aren't the most important thing—it is that you are healthy enough to enjoy your life, pursue your goals, and achieve your dreams. Perfect, just as you are.

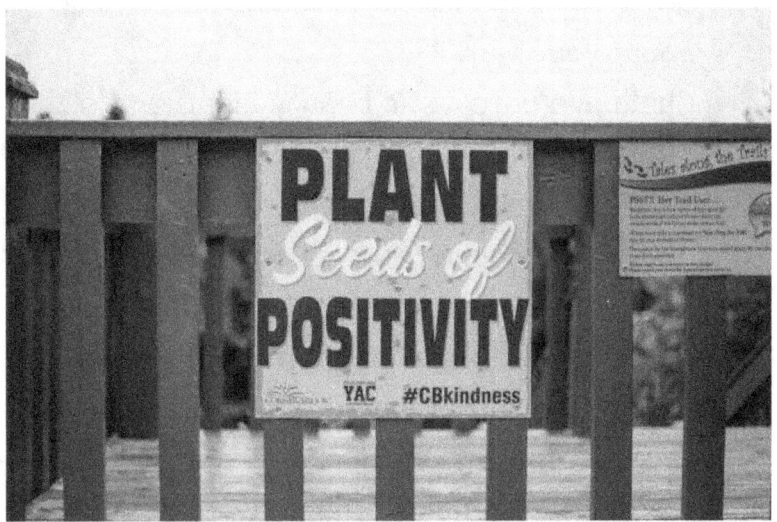

Practicing Body Positivity

Body positivity takes practice. You are changing habits and a mindset that you have carried for most of your life and are promoted and rewarded by society and the media. Breaking out of such a negative self-image and mindset will take effort, hard work, and a great deal of self-love and understanding. Here are a few ways you can practice body positivity to boost your mood, self-image, and your enjoyment of life.

- Practice self-compassion and show yourself kindness and understanding. Avoid being self-critical and engage in positive self-talk about your body.
- Challenge unrealistic beauty ideals and recognize that beauty is not limited to society's ideals. Don't compare yourself with other people—everyone's body is unique!
- Focus on functionality and shift your perception of your body to recognize and appreciate all the incredible things it is capable of and does. Celebrate your body's resilience, strengths, and uniqueness.
- Surround yourself with nothing but positive influences, such as body-positive social media accounts, communities, and friends and family who support you and promote your self-acceptance. Put uplifting posters or affirmations around your room or house to encourage positive thoughts.
- Diversify and control your media consumption. Purge your social media of posts and accounts that deal with dieting and weight loss or that promote negative

body image, and avoid anything that makes you feel bad about yourself. Watch films and TV with people and stories that make you feel seen and accepted and promote body positivity.

- Engage in activities you enjoy! Activities that bring you fulfillment and joy will help you focus on the experience rather than worrying about how your body looks while you do them. They'll also help you get out of your head, giving your mind a break.

- Set boundaries with people or situations that expose you to negative body talk or body shaming.

- Wear what makes you feel good! Ignore size labels—if it makes you feel good, that's all that matters! Ignore trends and instead find comfortable styles that make you feel confident. Pick colors and clothes that boost your mood and reflect who you are so you feel like you wear the clothes rather than hide beneath them. If you find shopping stressful or triggering, order clothes so you can try them on in the privacy and comfort of your own home, without judgment, or stuffy fitting rooms with lousy lighting and dirty mirrors.

- Practice mindfulness so you can be present in the moment and perceive your thoughts and feelings without judgment and negativity.
- Seek support from a therapist or counselor who specializes in body image issues.

20 Body Positive Affirmations

Affirmations are a great way to build up a body-positive attitude and show gratitude for your body. Vocalizing your appreciation for your body and high-lighting what you love about it boosts your mood and reinforces positive perceptions. You can also use affirmations on the go. Write them down on a piece of paper or your phone to carry with you, or you can record them to listen to when you feel trig-gered or particularly self-conscious. How you work with affirmations is up to you, so if you feel strange standing in front of the mirror talking to yourself, that's okay—find your own way! The important thing is to make your affirmations part of your daily routine to keep replenishing the good body vibes. Use the affirmations below to get you started, and over time, start adding your own.

1. I accept myself as I am right now.
2. My body deserves love, nourishment, and respect.
3. My body is my home, and I am grateful for it.
4. My body gives me life, and I am grateful for it.
5. I choose to be kind to my body.
6. My mind and my body are friends.
7. I am comfortable in my body.
8. My body gives me energy, vitality, and freedom.
9. My body can do incredible things.
10. My body is a source of strength and power.
11. It's okay for me to love myself.
12. My body is the perfect body for me.
13. I choose to love my body and be healthy.
14. My body gives the best hugs.
15. My body does not define me.
16. I measure my body in health, not numbers.
17. My body helps me do the things I enjoy most.
18. I eat to give my body love, energy, power, and support.
19. My body supports me through the hardest times.
20. I am worth my best efforts.

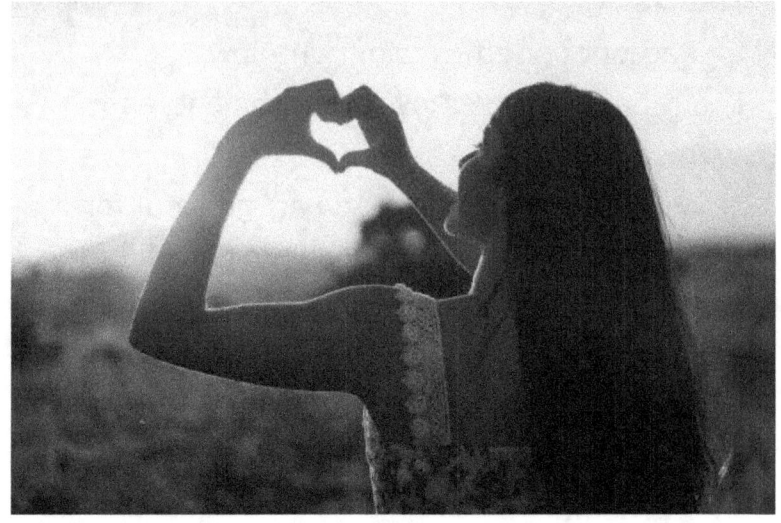

Step 7 Activity: Create Your Body Positivity Collage

Manifest body positivity by making a collage of images and words that help you feel confident and positive about your body. Display it somewhere you'll see it every day, or even beside a mirror, so that when you find yourself judging your appearance, you have a reminder right there to refocus your thoughts and push the negativity aside.

Learning to love and accept your body is hard work after feeling negative about it for so long. Seeing your body differently is a huge step, and treating it differently—with love and care—is just as important.

In the next chapter, we'll explore how you can boost your mind, body, and spirit with well-deserved, tender, loving self-care.

Chapter 8

Step 8 - Practicing Self-Care and Self-Love

You're on the path to recovery, but now you need to bring harmony and peace back into your mind and body by prioritizing self-care and self-love. Caring for yourself is a meaningful and rewarding task that helps you reconnect with your body in a compassionate and nurturing way—just what you need after so long of being unhappy with yourself.

Self-Care and Body Image Issues

Body dysmorphia prevents you from having a healthy relationship with yourself and can lead you to neglect your mental and physical needs and cause yourself harm. Self-care does the opposite. It promotes well-being by prioritizing and validating your needs and encouraging you to make positive changes to your habits and routines in order to improve your relationship with yourself. Self-care forces you to focus your attention inward and explore ways you can enhance your quality of life. It highlights how you can invest your time and energy in yourself rather than in worrying about other people or the world around you. It is a wonderful coping mechanism for when you feel anxious, stressed, overwhelmed, or experiencing many nega-tive thoughts. After a stressful day at work or school, anxious about people's opinions and your body, coming home to do some self-care is not only a reward for getting through the day but also an abso-lute necessity for healing and promoting a positive mindset. Self-care isn't just about pampering; it is about devoting time to inner and outer peace and harmony, nourishing your body and mind, and replenishing your energy.

Self-Care Activities

Self-care is one of the best ways to support your mental health and well-being, reduce your stress, and soothe anxiety. There are so many ways to incorporate self-care into your routine, many of them very affordable and accessible. You may not always feel like you have the time or energy to devote to self-care, but it's important that you try to make space for it in your life in any way you can, even if it is just five minutes of stretching, enjoying a cup of tea, or doing a face mask. Here are some great self-care activities that will fit easily into your lifestyle.

- **Meditation** is a great way to practice mindfulness and soothe your body and mind. It helps you tap into your thoughts and feelings and can take as long as you like. Try a short, guided meditation when you wake up or before bed to help you start and end the day on a positive note.
- **Exercise**: Get those endorphins flowing and your body moving, and you'll feel a rush of energy and a sense of achievement. Exercise has a lot of self-care benefits, allowing you to focus on your body's needs, give your mind a rest, and strengthen your body.
- Yoga is a perfect form of exercise for self-care. It stretches out all the stress and tension in your body, focuses your attention, and encourages you to connect with your body.

- **Get enough sleep:** Sleep is nourishing and energizing; it gives your body time to heal and restore itself and allows your mind to rest. A good sleep routine will help reduce anxiety and strengthen your body and mind.
- **Journaling** is a therapeutic and effective form of self-care that anyone can do! Use journal prompts to help you dig deeper into your thoughts and emotions, and try to keep your journaling practice regular.
- **Reading for pleasure**: Grab a cup of something hot and soothing, snuggle up with a blanket, and lose yourself in a good book.
- **Creative arts** make a great emotional outlet! Whether you like painting, drawing, writing poetry, dancing, or knitting, a creative hobby is a great way to express yourself and occupy your mind and attention.
- **Spend time in nature.** Nature has a wonderful healing effect on humans—fresh air, salty sea, green trees, blue sky, and sunshine all work wonders. Try to get outside for at least 20 minutes daily and be in nature, feeling and listening to it. Take a

walk or just sit on the grass and escape the confines of human society for a while.

- If nature is far away or you need a quick fix, get some houseplants and tend to them! They give back the energy you give them, plus they brighten up and boost the positive vibes of your home.
- **Deep abdominal breathing exercises** help to ground you and soothe anxiety, and you can do them anywhere at any time, absolutely free!
- **Spend quality time with loved ones** in comfortable and pleasant environments and doing activities you enjoy.
- **Disconnect from screens.** We're surrounded by screens almost all day, every day, so taking a break from them can help calm your mind and give you time to enjoy doing things you love without distractions. You could turn your phone off during your lunch break or set a "do not disturb" timer while practicing other forms of self-care to ensure you're not interrupted and distracted. Try to avoid screens entirely at least an hour before bed in order to get a good night's sleep.

- **Cooking and baking** distract your attention and keep your hands busy, and you get to enjoy the delicious fruits of your labor afterward!
- When you feel low, cooking and enjoying comfort food from your childhood can be an amazing way to practice self-care.
- **Take a hot bath** and really soak, letting the water draw out tension and negativity. Afterward, do a face mask, moisturize well, and put on a fluffy robe.
- **Laugh!** Watch comedies, play funny games, or read a funny book—laughter is the best medicine, after all!
- **Take breaks.** Be generous and allow yourself time to take a break when you feel overwhelmed. Just five minutes to reset and regroup can make a huge difference to your energy levels, productivity, and mental well-being.
- **Practice gratitude** to build a positive perception of your life.
- **Volunteering** is a rewarding and affirming activity that will make you feel good through helping others!
- **Listen to music...** and maybe dance around while you do!

- **Connect with animals!** Visit a local zoo or farm and interact with the animals. Animals can have a very calming energy and are just so cute you can't be sad around them.
- **Treat yourself** to a massage or spa day.
- **Eat well!** Have a dinner full of wholesome, fresh foods that will revitalize you and give your body a much-needed boost of vitamins and minerals.

You should also be sure to maintain a healthy work-life balance. While your job is inevitably going to be stressful sometimes, that stress is worth it if you enjoy what you do. Find time to decompress by yourself during the work day, don't take on more work than you can handle, and use your vacation days.

Most importantly, make sure you are attending to your basic needs. Getting enough sleep, eating well, drinking water, and exercising are the basics your body needs to function and support you through the day. No amount of self-care can make up for them!

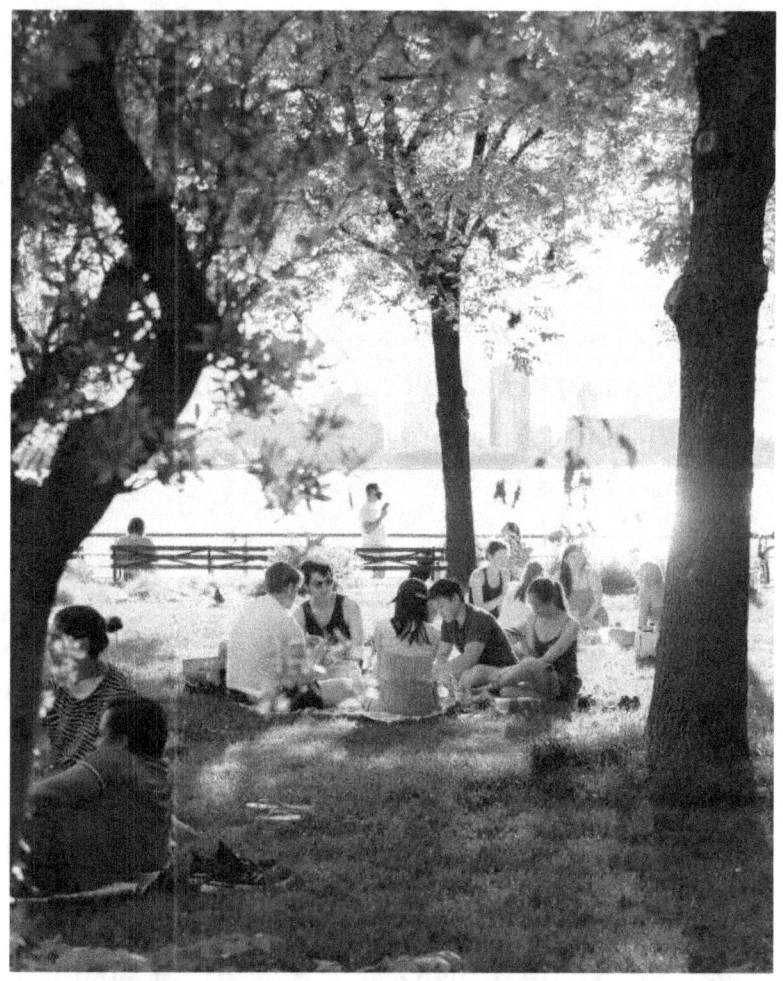

Cultivate Self-Love and Compassion

Self-love means showing yourself unconditional care, compassion, and understanding, which opens you up to appreciating yourself more and accepting who you are as you are. Self-love contributes to having good self-esteem because you feel happy people and influences and confident in yourself and know that you deserve good things. It also encourages you to take a positive view of yourself and the world. It motivates you to take action and put aside harmful behavior because you have a higher regard and respect for yourself and your abilities. This makes you more likely to take risks and challenge yourself, which gives you more opportunities for growth and self- discovery and can lead to a more prosperous and fulfilling life. Self-love also helps you stand up for yourself and say "no" to things that you don't want in your life, further removing sources of stress and increasing your resilience.

It takes effort and time to cultivate self-love, and it can feel uncomfortable at first, especially if you have spent a long time feeling negative about yourself. Self-love evolves over time through practice, intention, and changing mindsets and habits. There are many forms of self-love, and providing self-care is one of them. Others include:

- practicing self-compassion and kindness
- surrounding yourself with positive
- challenging negative self-talk
- setting healthy boundaries

- prioritizing your own needs
- celebrating and rewarding your achievements
- avoiding comparisons
- seeking out fulfilling and educational experiences
- practicing self-reflection and learning from past mistakes and problems
- embracing and using your uniqueness

In all these, the emphasis is on showing up for yourself and ensuring your decisions and actions serve your needs. You have to be your own priority, especially during your recovery from body image issues. Other people's thoughts, opinions, and actions may not always be in your best interests, so you have to keep a strong sense of self to understand who and what is worth your time and energy and who and what isn't. This is where boundaries come in.

Setting Boundaries and Saying No

Boundaries and Body Dysmorphia

Setting your own personal and interpersonal boundaries is essential for your recovery and mental health. Your energy should be focused on healing and recovery, not wasted on endeavors and people that only give you stress, anxiety, and negativity. Boundaries will help you control your environments and influences and help you focus on your priorities so that you can keep moving forward. Your boundaries should clearly show others how you want them to treat you and reinforce how you need to treat yourself.

Boundaries for body dysmorphia and eating disorders can involve having some difficult conversations with the most important people in your life. Your friends and family are likely to be supportive and eager to help but may be unaware that sometimes their words or actions are triggering. You'll need to explain what you need from them and call them out when they break a boundary once it is established, and while this can feel awkward and selfish, the people who genuinely love and support you will always strive to respect your needs and boundaries. Boundaries can help reinforce your relationship with people, too. It will help them be the best they can be for you and help you both avoid behaviors that inadvertently cause damage or that are triggering, meaning spending time with them is easier, and you feel more supported.

One of the toughest parts about setting boundaries, especially for people with anxiety, is saying "no," which comes with a fear of abandonment or an angry reaction. Saying "no" feels selfish and as though you are letting someone down, but if they are behaving in a way that breaches your boundaries or asking something of you that will compromise them, then you have to prioritize your health and needs and stand firm. They may have asked you out for dinner or want you to go shopping for outfits together. You know these activities will be triggering, and you'll spend the whole time anxious, afraid, and wishing you were anywhere else. In this moment, you have to think about what is best for yourself, and your stakes are higher than theirs. As lovely as it is that they want your company, you need to gently but firmly say "no." If you feel up to it and trust them, you can explain why but don't feel pressured to. Only ever say "yes" to activities, people, and situations in which you feel comfortable, supported, and positive.

Setting Boundaries for Your Mind, Body, and Other People

Self

Intrapersonal boundaries are just as important in your recovery as your boundaries with other people. You need to establish a sense of safety around yourself to move forward with strength and commitment, which begins within. Being aware of your symptoms and triggers will help you establish your personal boundaries and recognize what you need to do to protect your mental health and well-being. Firstly, you need to remove yourself from any abusive or traumatic environments or relationships, as these will hold your recovery back and continue to cause you harm even if you make progress in other areas. Working directly with a qualified therapist will help you identify the intrapersonal boundaries you need to establish, and they can also help you take the first difficult steps to cut off the people or things that are having a negative influence. You can then start to build boundaries that reinforce self-care practices across the most important areas: hygiene, nutrition, sleep, and rest for the body and mind.

Others

The boundaries you set for your interactions with others will help you to build the safe, reliable, and supportive relationships that you need during recovery. It is crucial that you create a supportive network around you, even when you feel incapable or like a burden. Positive influences in your life will make getting better a lot less stressful and keep you on track. You'll need to set both physical and mental or emotional boundaries.

- **Physical boundaries**

Your body and body image are in a vulnerable state during your recovery, and your physical boundaries are essential. Privacy, physical touch, and sexual behavior all fall under physical boundaries that you can set to ensure you feel safe and in control of your body. It's easy to see when these boundaries are being violated by you and by others, and you *must* let people know when they do so, or they will keep doing it. You'll fall into unhealthy behavioral patterns by accepting it to please them.

- **Mental/emotional boundaries**

These boundaries can be harder to recognize and set, and you'll need to be patient with people at first as they will also struggle to recognize them and when they are violating them. Boundary violations could be seemingly minor, like a friend sending you a social media post that triggers you, or they can be significant and detrimental, such as a family member commenting on or criticizing your appearance. The mental and emotional boundaries you set should cover:

- emotional needs
- feelings
- decision-making—choosing foods, clothes, activities, and other things may be stressful or triggering.
- time alone
- interests—things you were previously interested in may no longer be healthy or of interest.
- responsibilities
- roles within friend, family, and work group

It is important to note that **your boundaries shouldn't isolate you.** Instead, they should ensure you are surrounded by positive influences and people you can rely on and feel comfortable turning to when you need help and support. While your boundaries may limit your contact with certain people or activities, it is for a good reason, and in time and with recovery, you may slowly reconnect and reintegrate with them if they are still important to you.

Reinforcing Your Boundaries

Asking people to respect your boundaries is asking them to change their behavior, which can take time. They may slip up and forget, so you'll need to reinforce your boundaries. One way to do this is through the DEAR MAN technique, which breaks up a difficult conversation into parts so you can be clear and firm about your boundary needs.

- **Describe** your situation, the effect it is having on you, and what about it is making you anxious or stressed. Stick to the facts, and don't cast blame.

- **Express** your feelings about the situation. Use phrases like "I feel stressed because..." or "I feel angry when..."
- **Assert** yourself by asking clearly for what you need from them, for example, "I need you not to send me social media posts about dieting."
- **Reinforce** your needs by telling them why you need them to change their behavior and how it will help you and your relationship with them.
- Be **mindful**, focused, and firm in your point. If they try to challenge you, go back over the DEAR points patiently and clearly.
- **Appear** confident by speaking clearly and holding eye contact.
- **Negotiate** if necessary. If they aren't open to your needs, try to find alternative solutions, ask what they would prefer, and work around it.

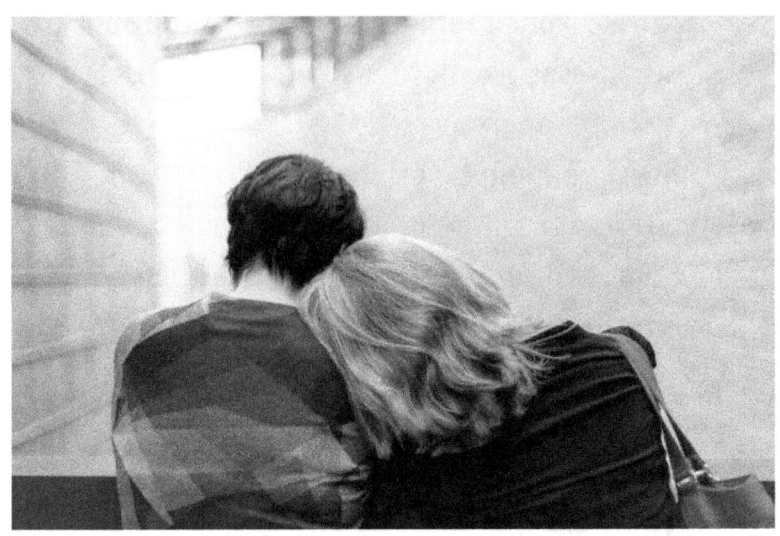

Step 8 Activity: Create Your Self-Care Routine

Routines are a fantastic tool for regulating your mental health. They help you organize your day, which soothes anxiety and makes sticking with your new habits easier. Incorporating self-care into your weekly or daily routine will make it a consistent and more rewarding practice.

Start by setting some weekly self-care goals that prioritize your recovery needs. If strengthening your body is a priority, try exercising three times a week for half an hour and doing a weekly meal plan on Sunday night. If you want to reduce your anxiety and soothe your mental health, you could set a consistent time to go to bed every night with a cup of chamomile tea or put in a 15-minute meditation or journaling session once a day to give both your body and mind a break. To put you in touch with your body, you might aim to pamper one part of yourself every evening with hand, foot, or face masks or take a hot bath every Sunday night to prepare your body for the next week.

Make sure you make time in your routine for self-care for your mind, body, and interests. Don't over-whelm yourself by filling up your routine too much straightaway—self-care should recharge you, not wear you out! Slowly incorporate self-care into your routine, using it to replace negative habits wherever you can.

Self-care helps to build you up but to stay strong in the face of setbacks and negativity; you'll need to learn to foster resilience in your everyday life. Growth and recovery take time, and resilience can help you bear the burdens that come with them so you can come out the other side stronger and more capable than ever. In the next chapter, you'll discover how to enhance your resilience and adopt a growth-focused mindset for the challenges ahead.

Chapter 9
Step 9 - Fostering Resilience and Growth

Resilience is a powerful life skill that you build up through experience, effort, and determination. Having a strong resilience makes a massive difference in your relationships, your mental health, and the way you live and approach your life. It is what helps you get back up when you're knocked down, what gives you the confidence to chase your dreams no matter the risk, and what gives you the courage to face the world and its challenges every day. For people with body dysmorphia and eating disorders, resilience plays an integral part in recovery and how they move forward through the rest of their lives.

Resilience and Body Dysmorphia

Resilience is your ability to adapt to and bounce back from challenges and setbacks. Resilient people are able to approach adversity with flexibility and persistence that allows them to bend and adjust rather than break, meaning that they can see through the bad times to enjoy the good times and rewards on the other side. Being resilient also allows you to learn and grow from the obstacles you meet and overcome rather than being beaten or demoralized by them. Your resilience is drawn from your inner strength, from skills, traits, and knowledge that you pick up throughout your life and throughout the hardships you face, which you can apply to situations when they arise to help you deal with them constructively and without suffering. Resilience gives you clarity about yourself in difficult times and situations. Without resilience, you are more prone to anxiety, feeling victimized, and becoming overwhelmed because you feel like you cannot draw on anything to help you.

There are many benefits to having resilience. Resilient people often feel more hopeful, optimistic, and satisfied about life because they feel capable of handling what it throws at them and experience lower stress and anxiety daily. Being resilient also means you can enjoy more emotional stability and build better communication skills so you feel comfortable and confident connecting with other people. It also means you use healthy coping mechanisms to deal with problems and develop good problem-solving skills that make handling stressful situations easier.

Resilience will be vital in moving forward through your recovery and your life beyond your struggles with body dysmorphia and eating disorders. It will help you cope with your triggers and foster growth that will overcome challenges that would formerly have set you back in your journey to wellness. Throughout your recovery, you'll encounter obstacles and challenging moments that you can either let hold you back or muster your resilience to push on and through. With each breakthrough and success—no matter how small it seems—your resilience increases, and in time, you'll find that things that used to scare or trigger you no longer hold as much power over you.

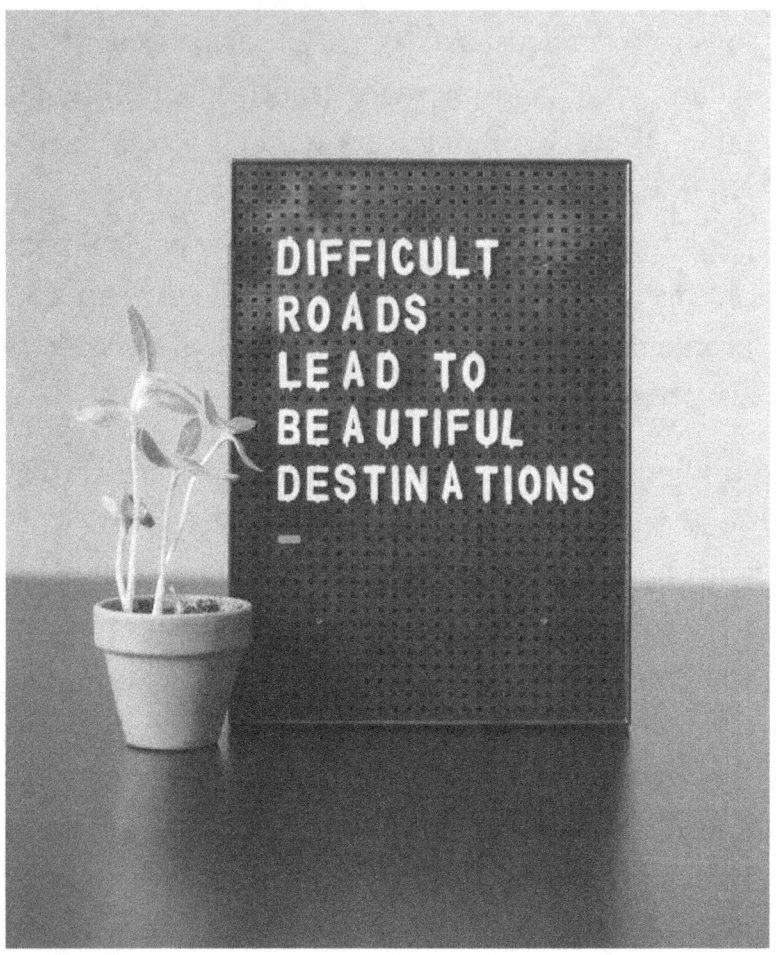

How to Build Your Resilience

Your resilience is drawn from every experience you've ever had. Still, instead of throwing yourself into a hundred new and scary situations in the name of building up your resilience, you can instead make these little, everyday changes to your habits and behavior that will imbue you with skills, mindsets, and goals that will boost your inner strength and your recovery.

- **Embrace a growth mindset.** We'll look closer at this one in the next section, but essentially, it means seeing setbacks and challenges as opportunities for you to grow and learn, encouraging yourself to see the positives in them rather than allowing them to negatively influence you and hold you back.
- **Build a supportive network** of strong relationships with people you trust and can rely on to do what is best for you and your recovery. A support system will alleviate some of your stress and open you up to more happiness, and you'll have people to fall back on in tough times. Remember to return the empathy you are extended in order to keep your relationships strong.
- **Practice self-compassion** and be understanding of your limitations and mistakes. Being gentle with yourself will help you bear your burdens.

- **Develop your problem-solving skills** by actively accepting tasks and putting yourself forward for challenging things. It's important to push yourself to prove that you are capable and to keep building your resilience skills by not avoiding things you fear you can't do.

- **Maintain perspective.** Remember that even when something seems overwhelming or impossible in the moment, time will pass, things will change, and in the end, it might not be as bad as you fear. Try to keep a sense of proportion when you panic, and look at challenges practically.

- **Set realistic and attainable goals and celebrate progress** no matter how small it seems! Goal setting—as we'll see in the next chapter—helps you focus on the future and look forward to a better life rather than dwelling on the past, and goals also give you purpose in the present, each day being a stepping stone to the future you aspire to.

- **Practice mindfulness** to regulate your thoughts and practice positive thinking. Negative thoughts are inevitable, but mindfulness will keep them from derailing your efforts by giving you the headspace to understand and correct them.

- **Prioritize physical health** as much as mental health. Good physical health plays a huge part in feeling good in your mind, too, so nourish and exercise your body as best you can and support it in being a safe, strong, and stable vessel for you during difficult times.
- **Be flexible and adaptable.** Resilience requires the flexibility of the mind to adapt when things don't go to plan. Change isn't easy or straightforward, but being open to it and adaptable to it will make your recovery a little easier and be extremely useful throughout your life.
- **Cultivate gratitude** and let your gratitude be known. It will bring positivity to your life and the lives of those who love and help you, and it will reinforce your sense of self-worth. You deserve all the good things you are grateful for!
- **Seek professional support if needed.** Turning to a professional for help is not an admission of failure—it takes a great deal of strength and self-confidence to open up about your struggles and ask for

help. A professional therapist will help you build and maintain your resilience and set and achieve your recovery goals.

- **Learn from adversity.** Things won't always go as you hope, and there will be times when you doubt yourself or feel incapable. In these times, you must step back, take a breath, and view the situation as a learning process. See where things went wrong, figure out how you can do things differently next time, and try again—*always* try again.

Developing a Growth Mindset

Cultivating a growth mindset means believing that your skills, talents, and intelligence develop and improve through overcoming adversity, putting in hard work, facing challenges, and accepting guidance from others. It is also believing that you have the ability and strength to grow, progress, and become a better version of yourself. People with a growth mindset see themselves and their abilities as constantly changing and evolving, and every challenge they face and overcome teaches them valuable lessons and increases their skillset so that they are better equipped and ready to deal with whatever is thrown at them next time. A growth mindset will give you confidence in yourself and the belief that your abilities, talents, and intelligence are ever-changing and able to improve, not fixed and restricted. This mindset stops you from limiting yourself and your goals and opens you up to a broader range of experiences and opportunities that can bring you fulfillment, success, and a better quality of life.

The very first step to developing a growth mindset is to approach challenges, fears, and the prospect of failure as opportunities for learning. This stops them from being so intimidating and makes you much more likely to pursue something, even if it scares you. One useful and positive way of viewing failure is to see it as a "not yet" instead of a "no" or "never." Try to recalibrate your thinking to allow for future growth by adding "yet" to negative thoughts, such as "I'm not good at this *yet*." Failure shouldn't stop you from trying again. Instead, it should highlight how you can improve and what more is required of you the next time around. There's no reason you shouldn't achieve your goal one day; you just weren't ready this time. Recognizing, understanding, and accepting your limitations will help to set realistic goals for yourself, which will help you avoid failure and also give you an idea of how much effort will be required of you from the start if you are to be successful.

Self-reflection is a potent tool for developing a growth mindset. You'll need to take the time to reflect on your successes and failures, recognize what you've learned on your journey to both, and lock in that knowledge for the future. Aim to do a reflective practice at the end of every day as a productive and important part of your recovery process. Another way to boost a growth mindset is to seek and learn from feedback. Criticism is always tough to take, but if you can see it as the chance to improve and show your skills rather than a personal attack, then you'll find more success and have a much more positive view of yourself and your endeavors. Don't rely on approval from others to give you worth or validate you, even if you hold them in high esteem and respect them. You determine your value with the goals you set and the efforts you make, and your reward should always be the knowledge that you have grown and learned rather than someone else's approval. This shouldn't stop you from extending your approval to others, though! Celebrating other people's success is an integral part of growth, and it should inspire you and teach you. Be curious about how they found success and see what you can learn from them, and stay curious in general about ways you can learn and grow.

Often, people praise success by labeling it with a trait such as being lucky or smart rather than praising the effort and actions it took to get there. Acknowledging your own and other's efforts is a tremendous growth mindset skill to have. It shows you appreciate the arduous journey and how much learning and work has been put in. You can turn this toward your achievements and make it part of your daily routine to praise and reward your efforts, especially if they are in pursuit of a goal that may take some time to achieve and that you need to stay motivated for—be your own cheerleader!

Step 9 Activity: Resilience Reflection

Write down and reflect on five times in your life that you have shown resilience and overcome a challenge. For each time, ask yourself these questions:

- What personal strengths helped you face the challenge and beat it?
- How did your success make you feel, and what were the rewards?

- What did you learn about yourself from the experience?
- How would you approach the same challenge now? Would you be successful again?

Use this reflective session to recognize and praise your past achievements. Show yourself that you have already overcome so much and you will do so again and that with every obstacle, you grow stronger and more resilient, even if you don't feel it right now.

Resilience is going to be an essential part of your recovery journey, especially because it will take all your resilience to keep pushing forward to achieve your personal goals when things don't go according to plan. In the next chapter, we'll explore how realistic and positive goal-setting plays a pivotal role in your recovery and how you can develop a clear and inspiring vision for your future beyond it.

Chapter 10
Step 10 - Embracing a Life of Purpose and Fulfillment

Beyond your recovery lies a life free of the burden of your condition, a life of possibilities and opportunities for joy, excitement, adventure, and connection. This may seem like a dream right now, far off and hard to imagine, but it is a very real future if you set it in motion now through goal-setting and a deeper understanding of what you value and desire most. Setting goals gives your recovery structure and focus and helps give you a sense of control over your life. Your goals will help you move forward positively through and after your recovery, giving you things to strive for that improve your life and bring you a sense of fulfillment and joy. By setting goals that support your values and passions, you are more likely to achieve them, and the simple act of setting goals drastically improves your chances of success.

Let's start by identifying what you want to pursue during and after your recovery.

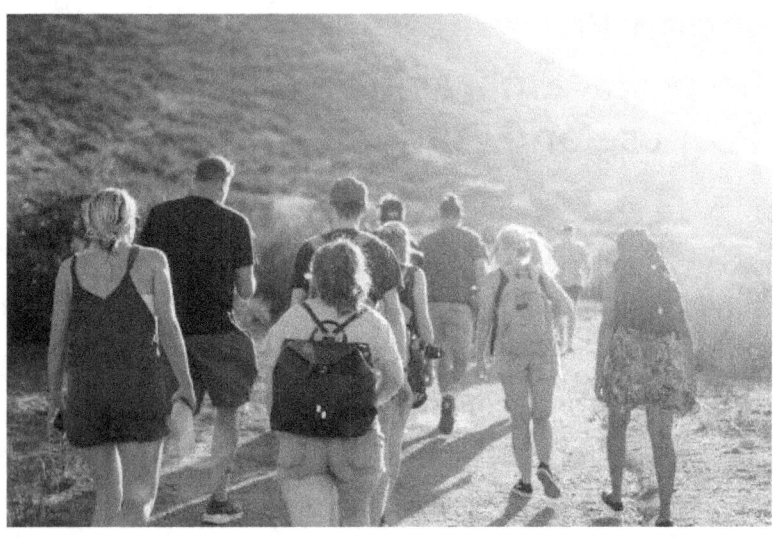

Discovering Your Personal Values and Passions

Personal Values and Eating Disorders

For as long as you have struggled with body dysmorphia or an eating disorder, your condition has exercised control over your values and interests, promoting damaging and negative "values" that govern your body image and self-image. To move forward in your recovery, you need to leave behind the old you and the old values that are doing more harm than good and rediscover what is truly impor-tant to you and your future health and happiness.

Values align with your beliefs, so if you believe negative things about yourself, your values will back up those beliefs and assign importance to things that validate the negative perceptions. An example of this is that many people with eating disorders highly value thinness or their ability to control their food intake because it aligns with their belief that their bodies must look a certain way in order to be acceptable. The values they hold here validate their belief and lead them to behave in a way that perpet-uates the problems associated with their condition. They need to change their values to reflect body-positive beliefs if they are going to be able to change their behavior for the better.

Your values provide you with a moral framework that helps you make decisions about what you want to spend your time and energy on. If you value your friendships, you're likely to spend a lot of time and energy on keeping them strong, and if you value getting good grades, you'll put a lot of time and effort into studying and revising. If your lifestyle or actions conflict with your values, you can experience intense feelings of shame, guilt, and dissatisfaction that severely impact your quality of life and cause your mental health to suffer. For people with eating disorders, this can create a vicious cycle. They might value their family's happiness so much that they hide their condition so as not to cause their family pain, but in doing so, make their condition worse, which then disrupts their home life and strains their relationship with their family. If your actions honor your values, you'll find that you can avoid these negative situations and build healthier habits and relationships built on honesty and under-standing.

Identifying Your Values and Passions

In order to set meaningful and inspiring goals that you are driven to achieve, you'll want to tailor them to your values and passions. This will keep you focused on the end goal and help you enjoy the journey more, even when it is tough. It will make your goals feel more worthwhile, rewarding, and exciting and will encourage you to set goals that challenge you and your growth. Most people's goals revolve around things like making more money or getting fit. However, for the benefit of your recovery and your continued health beyond it, your goals need to align with a more profound sense of self so that you continue to reap the rewards of your efforts long after you have achieved them and live a fulfilling life.

Your core values are unique to you and are influenced by your life experiences, upbringing, beliefs, and knowledge. You'll have core values across many areas of life, including ambition, charity, creativity, dependability, empathy, ethics, equality, freedom, fun, health, happiness, honesty, humor, individuality, intelligence, kindness, leadership, love, passion, performance, power, professionalism, relationships, risk, safety, success, wealth, and many more. Just reading that list, you probably had instinctual reactions or thoughts for each area, and these reactions hint at your values.

Here are some ways to dig deeper to understand the values and passions that drive your life and are worth aspiring to. There are no right or wrong answers here; your objective is to find your personal truth.

- **Self-reflection:** Take time often to reflect on your life experiences, things you find interesting, and things that bring you joy and a sense of fulfillment. Use self-reflection to understand your core beliefs and learn more about yourself.

- **Identify peak experiences** or the moments in your life that have felt like you've reached the top of a mountain— moments of feeling alive, free, and fulfilled. These experiences can show you what you feel most passionate about and the values that guided you to that moment.
- **Explore different activities** and try something new! New hobbies and interests can light a spark of joy you never knew was there, and trying new things may resonate with you unexpectedly and point you in a new direction and toward a new purpose.
- **Listen to your emotions** and let them guide you to activities that resonate positively with you. Take notice of how you feel during activities or experiences and how you feel when you engage with specific values. If you feel good, then your behavior is probably aligned with a passion or value that makes you happy.
- **Ask yourself these key questions** to get a deeper insight into what motivates you and what you value most about yourself and life:

  - What makes you excited to get out of bed in the morning?

○ What would you like to be remembered for?

○ Who do you consider a role model? Who is your hero? It could be a character from a book or film or someone real. What do you admire about them?

○ What hobbies bring you the most joy or excitement?

○ What kinds of movies or TV shows do you enjoy most, and what is it about them that you relate to?

○ What superpower would you most like to have? What does that superpower say about what you value or need in life?

- **Prioritize your values** by making a list of the qualities, morals, and principles that you value the most in yourself and in others. Then, use the top values to align your actions and decisions with them.

- **Experiment and adapt** to changes in your life and in your passions. Exploring a range of interests will expose you to new influences and ideas, keeping you open- minded and flexible.

- **Seek and follow inspiration.** Find role models, documentaries, TED talks, mentors, and books that will inspire you and align with your passions and values.

- **Volunteer or engage with your community.** Choose projects and activities that connect you to your interests and values. You could help in your local community or join a community that shares your passions, like a book club or local theater. You could also participate in events with the LGBTQ+ community or charities, like running a marathon to raise money.

- **Seek feedback** from people you love and trust about what they consider to be your strengths and passions. They see you differently and can offer a fresh and valuable perspective that you might not have considered.

- **Write a journal with the intention** of clarifying your thoughts and ideas and exploring your questions about your values. Look back through your journals to see if there are any common themes around values.

Setting Meaningful Goals

With your values and passions in mind, you can start to set goals that harness and channel their energy, bringing your life into alignment with your values and bringing you closer to the life you aspire to. Goals are important for everyone, giving you purpose and focus in your endeavors to achieve them and keeping you motivated through tough times, in the knowledge and hope that you will be rewarded with success. When you think about goals, you probably think of attaining milestones in life, "big picture" goals like getting a house, starting a family, going on a big vacation, or getting a promotion. Still, each of those goals is made up of many little, everyday goals, all of which act as stepping stones on the journey toward achieving the dream. These little, everyday goals are the most important ones of all, especially for people with body dysmorphia and eating disorders.

With any goal, the key to success is making the goal **specific, realistic, measurable,** and **time-relevant**. No goal can be achieved overnight. Instead, they require time and effort relative to the goal. If you are trying to achieve too much in too little time or without a clear idea of what is required of you, you'll inevitably end up failing to achieve it and being disheartened and discouraged. Small, achievable, and measurable goals will help you track your progress, lessen anxiety and pressure, and keep you moving forward a little at a time so you don't get overwhelmed or exhausted.

Eating Disorder Goals

Your recovery will depend on setting realistic, achievable, and reasonable goals for yourself. Such goals that won't overwhelm you or drain you, and that will keep you motivated and on track to recovery. In eating disorder recovery, goals provide stability, focus, and a healthy sense of control over your time and energy. Your recovery goals should reinforce positive behavior patterns and challenge disordered behaviors associated with food, exercise, and weight. Your goals should also help you develop healthier coping mechanisms so that you don't simply replace one unhealthy behavior with another. These goals will also help you maintain good habits and help you feel that you are making gradual and measurable progress, which will boost your confidence and self-image.

When setting your recovery goals, avoid using words like "always" and "never," as these enforce the idea of perfectionism and an "all or nothing" mindset that doesn't encourage healthy habits or thought patterns. You want to keep some flexibility in your goals that allows for bad days or the unexpected rather than setting defined terms that mean success or failure, which are the only options. Your goals should be tailored to your condition, circumstances, and lifestyle. Your goals should challenge you just enough to ensure progress but not so much that they become too much, and you slip back into old, negative habits that are easier and feel "safer." Be honest with yourself—and your therapist—about your fears and limitations when goal-setting, and remember that what works for someone else may not be suitable for you—your recovery is your own unique, personal journey.

Twelve Tiny Recovery Goals

Here are some little recovery goal ideas that you can implement right away into your daily routine and start on the track to your bigger goals:

1. Do 15 minutes of journaling or mindfulness meditation every morning this week.
2. Follow your healthy meal plan for three days in a row.
3. Call a loved one when you feel triggered.
4. Spend 10 minutes a day on self-care.
5. Attend a recovery support group once a week for a month.
6. Unfollow three social media accounts that you find triggering.
7. Write and speak a positive affirmation every morning.
8. Treat yourself once a week to something outside your comfort zone, whether that's dessert or new clothes.
9. Get rid of your scale!
10. Start a new hobby.
11. Spend an hour three days this week on a hobby or interest that makes you happy.
12. Go for a walk in nature twice this week.

These are all small but very attainable goals that take minimal effort but can make a huge difference in your journey toward your ultimate goal of recovery. None of these little goals require you to go out of your way to change anything huge about your life, but they do reinforce positive behavior and coping mechanisms that, in time, will become habits. Not achieving any one of these won't be the end of the world. You won't have "failed," and it won't set you back in your recovery—it will just be something to make a little time for tomorrow. Be gentle with yourself, as new habits and goals take time to embrace.

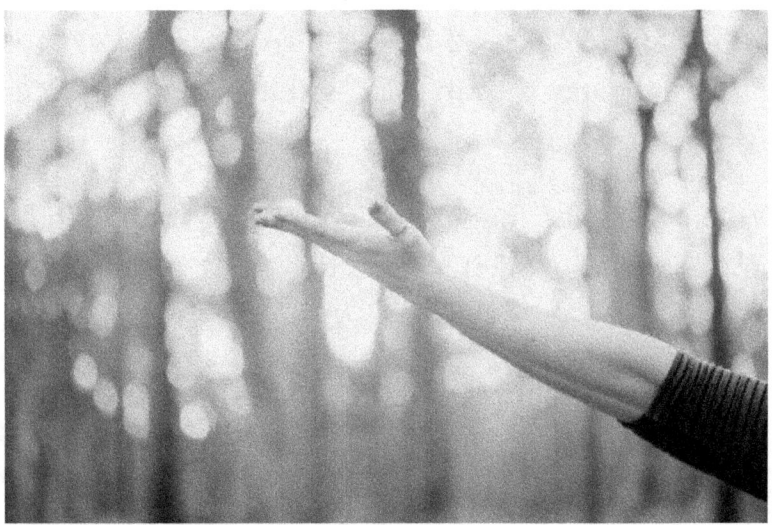

Personal and Life Goals

Beyond your recovery, you have a long life of personal goals waiting to be achieved. Setting these goals during your recovery will help you see beyond your condition and toward a bright future full of adventure, happiness, and success. Life goals tend to fall under either long-term or short-term goals and usually revolve around personal, professional, financial, educational, and social goals. Goal-setting helps you identify what you strive to accomplish in life and gives you an idea of how you can go about it with focus and purpose rather than just vague and unrealistic, hoping that everything falls into place. It can help you build a framework for your life that includes everything you enjoy and value and motivates you to succeed by making clear the rewards you can expect from successfully achieving your goals.

When setting your **personal goals,** you should consider three key things:

1. **Your passions:** Do your goals allow you to explore and enjoy your passions? Will you be passionate about pursuing your goal as well as the result of it?
2. **Goal control:** You should be able to control your journey to achieving your goal as much as possible. Goals that depend on luck, chance, external factors, and other people's efforts are likely to fail.
3. **The ideal outcome:** What would your life look like ideally if you achieved your goal? What would be the price and reward of

success, and will they be worth the journey and sacrifices to come?

Top Goal Tips

Use these tips to hone your goals and make them as achievable as possible:

- **Make SMART goals:** SMART goals are a method of goal-setting that boosts your chances of success by setting out your goal in clear terms.

  - **Specific:** Your goal needs to have a specific aim—anything too broad or vague, and the risk of failure increases!
  - **Measurable:** You need to be able to measure when the goal is a success or completed so that you know when you are close to success and have achieved your aim.
  - **Attainable:** Your goal should be a realistic option for you based on your abilities, circumstances, time, and any other data.

- ○ **Relevant:** Your goal should be relevant to your life and aims—you don't want to waste time and energy on a goal that, in the long run, will have no real impact or use!
- ○ **Time-bound:** Goals should always be given a time frame or deadline that is realistic. If they are too far in the future, goals can be easily put off or forgotten. If they are too soon, they become a burden and a cause of anxiety and stress. Give yourself time in relation to the complexity of the goal.

- **Write your goals down**; don't just keep them in your head! Writing them down makes them more real—a physical admission of your intentions.
- **Make your goals visible** with mood boards, notes on the fridge or bathroom mirror, or inspiring pictures or quotes at the office. This will keep your goal in the front of your mind and keep motivating you every time you see it.
- **Break them down** into smaller, less overwhelming steps. You could draw a goal ladder, with your ultimate goal at the top

and smaller goals on each rung leading up to it. This will also help you plan each step of the journey and track your progress.

- **Check your perspective.** It's easy to become goal-obsessed, and this can lead to burnout or to you abandoning other goals and responsibilities in favor of your obsession. Remember that your goal is just one part of your life, and that balance is key. Take breaks when you need them, be kind to yourself, and don't try to rush anything.
- **Recognize obstacles** and prepare for them as best you can. Pursuing your goal will inevitably mean facing challenges, so look ahead and try to imagine what some might be so that you can prepare for them now. This will make them less intimidating and scary when they happen.
- **Keep yourself accountable** by letting other people know about your aims and encouraging them to track your progress with you. This will keep you focused and consistent in your efforts, and they'll be there to celebrate with you at the end!
- **Reflect, adapt, and adjust** when things don't work out. It's okay not to achieve your goal—maybe you didn't have enough time,

or the unexpected happened. Step back, take a breath, and reflect on where things went wrong and what you can change or adjust to make the goal more achievable next time. Replan and start again.

Step 10 Activity: Your Life Vision Board

With your goal-setting mindset switched to the max, it's time to look to the future and your life beyond recovery. For this activity, make a vision board of what you want your life to look like post-recovery. Fill the board with dreams, goals, and inspirations. You can include people or characters you admire, places you want to visit or live in, jobs or hobbies you want to try, and motivational quotes. Find space for positive self-talk, writing yourself notes that begin with "I will..." When the board is done, put it somewhere you'll see it every day, and let it be a beacon of light throughout your recovery, a glimpse into the beautiful future that awaits you. You can keep adding to it, too—you and your future constantly evolve!

Before You Start on Your Journey...

If this book has helped you overcome anxiety about body image and disordered thoughts, and inspired you to unlock everything you need to embrace your body (and yourself) as you are, we hope you can do us a favor and leave a quick review on Amazon.

Share your thoughts on the 10 simple steps and let them know how it made you feel. We would love to hear how this easy-to-follow routine impacted you and helped you to form a whole new mindset, one embodied by body positivity and neutrality.

WANT TO HELP OTHERS?

Thank you for your support. We are so looking forward to someone reading your words and deciding that this is the day they will take their health into their hands and put an end to bad habits standing in the way of success.

Scan the QR code below

Conclusion

Recovery from body image issues, body dysmorphia, and eating disorders is a long road, full of challenges and obstacles but also opportunities for incredible growth and discovery. Your journey through this book has given you valuable skills and habits that will help you far beyond these pages, and you have a lifetime ahead to enjoy the rewards of the hard work that has been asked of you. You've done an amazing job so far. You've delved deep into difficult questions, you've explored hidden fears and harsh truths, and, step-by-step, you've built up a stronger and healthier connection with yourself and your body. You've learned to be kind to yourself and to treat yourself with care and compassion. A bright future awaits you, where you can wear and eat what you like without fear or anxiety and where your goals and dreams revolve around love and fun, not how you look.

There will be tough days when no matter how hard you've worked or how well you've stuck to your new routines and habits, you feel unmotivated or as though you've missed a step and fallen behind in your recovery. On these days, remember how far you have come and how hard you have tried, and don't let one bad day dictate your success and deprive you of many more good days. The only way to fail is to give up trying, and you are worth so much more than that! When you feel down and struggle to get back up, return to this book and the activities and start over if you have to. This book will always be here to remind you of how strong and capable you are, how difficult what you are dealing with is, and how amazing you are for not letting it rule you anymore.

Even though this book is ending, your journey has only just started. This is your time now, time to take back control of your life, time to refocus and recon-nect and restore power to your body and mind. You have a wealth of healthy habits, positive influences, and self-knowledge at your disposal, ready to unleash on the world and your goals, and there's nothing to stop you anymore. Go out into the world with confidence and compassion, and enjoy every reward you've earned!

References

Ackerman, C. E. (2018, July 20). *What is self-compassion and self-love? (Definition, quotes + books)*. Positive Psychology. https://positivepsychology.com/self-compassion-self-love/

ANAD. (2021). *Eating disorder statistics | general & diversity stats*. National Association of Anorexia Nervosa and Associated Disorders; ANAD. https://anad.org/eating-disorders-statistics/

BDD Foundation. (n.d.). *Famous people with BDD*. Body Dysmorphic Disorder Foundation. Retrieved October 14, 2023, from https://bddfoundation.org/information/more-about-bdd/famous-people-with-bdd/

Better Health Channel. (2015, September 18). *Stigma, discrimination and mental illness*. Better Health Channel; Victoria State Government. https://www.betterhealth.vic.gov.au/health/servicesandsupport/stigma-discrimination-and-mental-illness

Bettino, K. (2021, June 2). *What's CBT and is it right for me?* Psych Central. https://psychcentral.com/lib/in-depth-cognitive-behavioral-therapy#is-it-right-for-me

Brennan, D. (2021, March 29). *How does mental health affect physical health?* WebMD. https://www.webmd.com/mental-health/how-does-mental-health-affect-physical-health

Buchwald, N. (2020, July 3). *5 emotional regulation skills*. Manhattan Mental Health Counseling. https://manhattanmentalhealthcounseling.com/5-emotional-regulation-skills/

Center for Discovery. (2018, January 4). *18 eating disorder recovery goals for 2018*. Center for Discovery. https://centerfordiscovery.com/blog/18-eating-disorder-recovery-goals-2018/

Centers for Disease Control and Prevention. (2019). *Improving your eating habits*. Centers for Disease Control and Prevention. https://www.cdc.gov/healthyweight/losing_weight/eating_habits.html

Coelho, S., & Smith, J. (2013, June 13). *Benefits of self-compassion: 7 benefits and how to practice*. Psych Central. https://psychcentral.com/blog/practicing-self-compassion-when-you-have-a-mental-illness

Cooks-Campbell, A. (2022, May 26). *What self-love truly means and ways to cultivate it*. BetterUp. https://www.betterup.com/blog/self-love

Damin, R. (2021, October 25). *How to cultivate self-love*. Intuitive Healing Psychotherapy Practice . https://www.intuitivehealingnyc.com/blog/2021/10/17/how-to-cultivate-self-love

Deering, S. (2023, January 25). *20 easy ways to practice self-care each and every day*. Today. https://www.today.com/life/inspiration/self-care-ideas-rcna65285

Eatough, E. (2021a, July 15). *10 tips to set goals and achieve them*. BetterUp. https://www.betterup.com/blog/how-to-set-goals-and-achieve-them

Eatough, E. (2021b, October 6). *Why you need a self-care plan (and 5 ways to get started)*. BetterUp. https://www.betterup.com/blog/self-care-plan

EDCare. (2021, August 31). *Boundaries in eating disorder recovery: What, why, and how*. EDCare. https://eatingdisorder.care/boundaries-and-eating-disorder-recovery/

Eddins, R. (2020, October 7). *Emotional regulation skills to cope with difficult emotions: 7 skills to practice today*. Eddins Counseling Group. https://eddinscounseling.com/emotion-regulation-coping-skills/

Ekern, B. (2019, October 7). *Building resiliency to improve the recovery skills of daughters who have eating disorders*. Eating

Disorder Hope. https://www.eatingdisorderhope.com/blog/improve-daughters-resilience-eating-disorder-treatment

Ekern, J. (2019). *Effective coping skills used in eating disorder recovery.* Eating Disorder Hope. https://www.eatingdisorderhope.com/recovery/self-help-tools-skills-tips/effective-coping-for-eating-disorders

Foy, C. (2022, October 13). *Unrealistic beauty standards and mental health.* FHE Health – Addiction & Mental Health Care. https://fherehab.com/learning/beauty-standards-mental-health#:

FutureLearn. (2022, April 25). *What is a growth mindset and how can you develop one?* FutureLearn. https://www.futurelearn.com/info/blog/general/develop-growth-mindset

Germer, C. K. (2009). *The mindful path to self-compassion: Freeing yourself from destructive thoughts and emotions.* Guilford.

Grouport. (2023, August 28). *Empowering self-reflection with cognitive behavior therapy journal prompts: Ideas and examples.* Grouport Therapy. https://www.grouporttherapy.com/blog/cbt-journal-prompts

Harvard Health Publishing. (2013, June 27). *The power of self-compassion.* Harvard Health; Harvard Medical School. https://www.health.harvard.edu/healthbeat/the-power-of-self-compassion#:

Harvard School of Public Health. (2017, November 20). *Make exercise a daily habit – 10 tips.* The Nutrition Source; Harvard School of Public Health. https://www.hsph.harvard.edu/nutritionsource/2013/11/04/making-exercise-a-daily-habit-10-tips/

Health Direct. (2023, May 24). *Exercise and mental health.* Health Direct . https://www.healthdirect.gov.au/exercise-and-mental-health#:

Holland, M. (2022, November 18). *15 common anxiety triggers &*

how to cope with them. Choosing Therapy. https://www.choosingtherapy.com/anxiety-triggers/

Indeed Editorial Team. (2022, August 8). *6 steps to discover your core values*. Indeed. https://www.indeed.com/career-advice/career-development/discover-core-values

Jaramillo, S. (2021, December 6). *Eating disorder recovery meal plans*. Peace & Nutrition. https://peaceandnutrition.com/eating-disorder-recovery-meal-plans/

Karst, N. (2018, July 30). *Who am I without anorexia? Finding purpose, meaning, and your true self in recovery – part 9*. Eating Disorder Hope. https://www.eatingdisorderhope.com/blog/personal-values-spirituality-your-true-self-recovery-part-9

Katz Leon, S. (2012, January 30). *Body image issues and healthy boundaries*. Good Therapy. https://www.goodtherapy.org/blog/body-image-issues-and-healthy-boundaries-013012

Klynn, B. (2021, June 22). *Emotional regulation: Skills, exercises, and strategies*. BetterUp. https://www.betterup.com/blog/emotional-regulation-skills

Kristenson, S. (2023, April 4). *71 body positive affirmations to feel your best*. Happier Human. https://www.happierhuman.com/body-positive-affirmations/

Lieberman, C. (2017, December 14). *What body dysmorphia actually feels like*. Talkspace. https://www.talkspace.com/blog/what-body-dysmorphia-actually-feels-like/

Malmon, A. (2022). *Self-care*. Active Minds. https://www.activeminds.org/about-mental-health/self-care/

Manwaring, J. (2022, October 3). *Why is being self-aware important for your mental health?* Alvarado Parkway Institute. https://apibhs.com/2022/10/03/why-is-being-self-aware-important-for-your-mental-health

Mayo Clinic. (2017, July 14). *Eating disorder treatment: Know your options*. Mayo Clinic. https://www.mayoclinic.org/diseases-

conditions/eating-disorders/in-depth/eating-disorder-treat
ment/art-20046234

Mayo Clinic. (2021, December 16). *Fitness program: 5 steps to get started*. Mayo Clinic. https://www.mayoclinic.org/healthy-lifestyle/fitness/in-depth/fitness/art-20048269#:

Mayo Clinic. (2022a, July 14). *Resilience: Build skills to endure hardship*. Mayo Clinic. https://www.mayoclinic.org/tests-proce
dures/resilience-training/in-depth/resilience/art-20046311#:

Mayo Clinic. (2022b, December 13). *Body dysmorphic disorder - symptoms and causes*. Mayo Clinic. https://www.mayoclinic.
org/diseases-conditions/body-dysmorphic-disorder/symp
toms-causes/syc-20353938

McCabe, M. (2018, December 17). *How to set recovery goals in the beginning*. Angie Viets - Inspired Recovery. https://www.
angieviets.com/articles/how-to-set-recovery-goals-in-the-beginning

Mental Health Foundation. (2022, February 18). *Physical health and mental health*. Mental Health Foundation. https://www.
mentalhealth.org.uk/explore-mental-health/a-z-topics/physi
cal-health-and-mental-health#:

Metcalf, E. (2019, November 1). *My path to accepting mental illness*. NAMI: National Alliance on Mental Illness. https://
www.nami.org/Blogs/NAMI-Blog/November-2019/My-Path-to-Accepting-Mental-Illness

Mind. (2022, July). *Body dysmorphic disorder (BDD)*. Mind.org.uk. https://www.mind.org.uk/information-support/types-of-mental-
health-problems/body-dysmorphic-disorder-bdd/about-bdd/

Mind Tools Content Team. (2022a). *Personal goal setting*. Mind Tools. https://www.mindtools.com/a5ykiuq/personal-goal-
setting

Mind Tools Content Team. (2022b). *What are your values?* Mind Tools. https://www.mindtools.com/a5eygum/what-are-your-
values

Mind Tools Content Team. (2023). *Developing resilience.* Mind Tools. https://www.mindtools.com/ao310a2/developing-resilience

Mindful. (2019, June 12). *How to meditate for anxiety.* Mindful. https://www.mindful.org/mindfulness-meditation-anxiety/

Mizock, L. (2017, February 27). *Five tips to accept a mental health problem.* Psychology Today. https://www.psychologytoday.com/us/blog/the-health-women/201702/five-tips-accept-mental-health-problem

Morand, M. (2019). *Renfrew professional webinar: Navigating higher levels of care - tools for treatment transitions.* Eating Disorder Hope. https://www.eatingdisorderhope.com/recovery/self-help-tools-skills-tips/goal-setting

National Institute of Mental Health. (2022, December). *Caring for your mental health.* National Institute of Mental Health. https://www.nimh.nih.gov/health/topics/caring-for-your-mental-health

Neff, K. (2015a, February 23). *Exercise 2: Self-Compassion break.* *Self-Compassion.* https://self-compassion.org/exercise-2-self-compassion-break/

Neff, K. (2015b, February 23). *Exercise 4: Supportive touch.* *Self-Compassion.* https://self-compassion.org/exercise-4-supportive-touch/

Nussbaum, A. (2020, August 1). *Goal setting in eating disorder recovery.* BALANCE Eating Disorder Treatment Center. https://balancedtx.com/blog/goal-setting-in-eating-disorder-recovery

ODPHP. (2015). *How to build a healthy eating pattern.* Office of Disease Prevention and Health Promotion. https://health.gov/sites/default/files/2019-10/DGA_Healthy-Eating-Pattern.pdf

Pedersen, T. (2016, May 17). *Triggers: What they are, how they form, and what to do.* Psych Central. https://psychcentral.com/lib/what-is-a-trigger#:

Pedersen, T. (2022, October 26). *Therapy for eating disorders:*

Treatment options to consider. Psych Central. https://psych central.com/eating-disorders/therapy-for-eating-disorders

Pedersen, T. (2023, February 27). *Social media and body image: What's the link?* Psych Central. https://psychcentral.com/health/how-the-media-affects-body-image

Petre, A. (2022, April 11). *Learn about 6 common types of eating disorders and their symptoms.* Healthline. https://www.health line.com/nutrition/common-eating-disorders#-5.-Rumination-disorder

Quinlan, K. (2020, June 19). *Ep. 153: A self-compassion letter - therapy for OCD & eating disorders.* Kimberley Quinlan - Therapy & Counseling for OCD & Eating Disorders. https://kimberleyquinlan-lmft.com/ep-153-a-self-compassion-letter/#:

Raypole, C. (2020, November 13). *Emotional triggers: Definition and how to manage them.* Healthline. https://www.healthline.com/health/mental-health/emotional-triggers

Rivera, A. (2022, November 21). *Setting boundaries in eating disorder recovery.* ACUTE. https://www.acute.org/blog/setting-boundaries-eating-disorder-recovery

Robinson, L., Segal, J., & Smith, M. (2023, February 28). *The mental health benefits of exercise.* Help Guide. https://www.helpguide.org/articles/healthy-living/the-mental-health-bene fits-of-exercise.htm

Sutton, J. (2022, January 28). *How to use mindfulness therapy for anxiety: 15 exercises.* Positive Psychology. https://positivepsy chology.com/mindfulness-for-anxiety/

Swaim, E. (2022, December 22). *What's resilience? Benefits and tips for "bouncing back" after hardship.* Healthline. https://www.healthline.com/health/mental-health/what-is-resilience

Tewari, A. (2022, July 14). *100 powerful body positive affirmations for loving your body.* Gratitude. https://blog.gratefulness.me/body-positive-affirmations/

Thurmond, N. (2019). *Healing from trauma and setting boundaries in relationships*. Eating Disorder Hope. https://www.eatingdisorderhope.com/treatment-for-eating-disorders/co-occurring-dual-diagnosis/trauma-ptsd/healing-from-trauma-and-setting-boundaries-in-relationships

Vogel, K. (2022, May 6). *The 3 basic principles of cognitive behavioral therapy*. Psych Central. https://psychcentral.com/pro/the-basic-principles-of-cognitive-behavior-therapy#cbt-techniques

West, M. (2022, April 29). *Body positivity movement: Benefits, drawbacks, vs. body neutrality*. Medical News Today. https://www.medicalnewstoday.com/articles/body-positivity

Wooll, M. (2021, July 26). *A growth mindset is a must-have — these 13 tips will grow yours*. BetterUp. https://www.betterup.com/blog/growth-mindset

Image References

AllGo An App For Plus Size People. (16 Nov. 2019) *"Plus Size People at Work in Bright, Open Office Workplace"* [Image]. Unsplash. unsplash.com/photos/four-persons-sitting-on-chairs-near-window-during-daytime-1GEsAeUv5dU. Accessed Oct. 2023.

Burke, Jennifer (2 Aug. 2016). *"Person's Left Hand Wrapped in Tape Measure"* [Image]. Unsplash , unsplash.com/photos/persons-left-hand-wrapped-by-tape-measure-ECXB0YAZ_zU. Accessed Oct. 2023.

Busing, Hannah. (20 Feb. 2020). *"Girl Friends Hands Piled Together,"* [Image]. Unsplash. unsplash.com/photos/person-in-red-sweater-holding-babys-hand-Zyx1bK9mqmA. Accessed Oct. 2023.

Dahl, Mason. (21 June 2020). *"People Sitting on Green Grass near Trees"* [Image]. Unsplash. unsplash.com/photos/people-sitting-on-green-grass-field-near-green-trees-during-daytime--7AxXbZekDE. Accessed Oct. 2023.

David, Jackson. (17 Aug. 2019). *"Heart Hands Woman"* [Image]. Pexels. www.pexels.com/photo/shallow-focus-photo-of-woman-in-white-thick-strap-top-showing-heart-hand-gesture-2810210/. Accessed Oct. 2023.

Dryden, James. (16 Feb. 2020). *"Post-It Note Person"* [Image]. Unsplash. unsplash.com/photos/person-in-yellow-shirt-with-white-printer-paper-ZDG2n7Qg3nI. Accessed Oct. 2023.

Du Preez, Priscilla. (9 Nov. 2020). *"Couple Holding Hands"* [Image]. Unsplash. unsplash.com/photos/person-in-black-long-sleeve-shirt-holding-babys-feet-aPa843frIzl. Accessed Oct. 2023.

Du Preez, Priscilla. (6 Mar. 2019). *"Woman Wearing Gray Jacket"* [Image]. Unsplash. unsplash.com/photos/woman-wearing-gray-jacket-F9DFuJoS9EU. Accessed Oct. 2023.

Ello. (1 Dec. 2020). *"Meal Prep Salmon"* [Image]. Unsplash. unsplash.com/photos/sliced-lemon-on-white-plastic-container-94KPme-Ibb4. Accessed Oct. 2023.

Grainger, Natalie. (18 Dec. 2016). *"Person Lifting Her Hand"* [Image]. Unsplash. unsplash.com/photos/tilt-shift-lens-photography-of-person-lifting-hand-8uB5kFKWWkk. Accessed Oct. 2023.

Kulikova, Klara. (17 Mar. 2021). *"Woman Covering Her Breast with Her Hand"* [Image]. Unsplash. , unsplash.com/photos/woman-covering-her-breast-with-her-hand-TcUfF24fUMY. Accessed Oct. 2023.

Mangano, Jessica. (17 July 2020). *"Journaling beside a Lake"* [Image]. Unsplash. unsplash.com/photos/person-writing-on-white-paper-NUQtVifTqs4. Accessed Oct. 2023.

Marea Wellness. (22 June 2023). *"Embracing Inner Peace and Discovering Harmony through the Transformative Practice of*

Meditation." [Image]. Unsplash.unsplash.com/photos/a-group-of-people-doing-yoga-in-a-park-nmHSysCA_Mk. Accessed Oct. 2023.

Mclean, Eric. (21 Aug. 2021). *"Pink and White Wooden Signage"* [Image]. Unsplash. unsplash.com/photos/pink-and-white-wooden-signage-EoVoOCNf8nc. Accessed Oct. 2023.

Nik. (11 June 2018). *"Difficult Roads Lead to Beautiful Destinations"* [Image]. Unsplash. unsplash.com/photos/difficult-roads-lead-to-beautiful-destinations-desk-decor-z1d-LP8sjuI. Accessed Oct. 2023.

Olinger, Hannah. (7 Feb. 2018). *"Journaling over Coffee"* [Image]. Unsplash. unsplash.com/photos/a-person-writing-on-a-piece-of-paper-with-a-pen-8eSrC43qdro. Accessed Oct. 2023.

Popovic, Milan. (21 May 2018). *"Woman Sitting on Cliff Overlooking Mountains"* [Image]. Unsplash. unsplash.com/photos/woman-sitting-on-cliff-overlooking-mountains-during-daytime-Zf0-90SpDD0. Accessed Oct. 2023.

Porter, Luke. (10 Sept. 2018). *"People Walking on Dirt Road in Daytime"* [Image]. Unsplash. unsplash.com/photos/people-walking-on-dirt-road-near-mountain-during-daytime-NEqEC7qa9FM. Accessed Oct. 2023.

Tonn, Motoki. (19 Oct. 2019). *"Mindful Walk with Anne Marie"* [Image]. Unsplash.unsplash.com/photos/boy-leaning-back-on-tree-X00q3RXcyZ4. Accessed Oct. 2023.

Transly Translation Agency. (14 Oct. 2018). *"Woman Rests Her Head on Shoulder"* [Image]. Unsplash. unsplash.com/photos/a-woman-rests-her-head-on-another-persons-shoulder-KQfxVDHGCUg. Accessed Oct. 2023.

www.ingramcontent.com/pod-product-compliance
Lightning Source LLC
Chambersburg PA
CBHW060922120626
46557CB00003B/844